Praise for Upg

"*Interesting and engaging. Having tasted many of Deirdre's imaginative recipes, I can't wait for the recipe book to follow!*"

– Dr. Peter A. Purpura

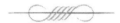

"*It's the bible for good nutrition, with excellent specifics and tips on all facets of the food industry and nutrition.*"

– Dr. Aashish D Dadarwala, Doctor of Osteopathic Medicine, Attending Faculty at Beth Israel Family Medicine Residency, New York, New York.

UPGRADE YOUR LIFE
ONE BITE AT A TIME

A RESOURCE GUIDE TO EATING YOUR WAY TO
PERFECT HEALTH & IDEAL WEIGHT

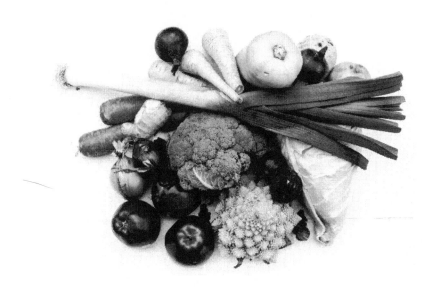

DEIRDRE VENTURA

To contact the publisher, visit www.THRHospitality.com.
To contact the author, visit www.HealthyLivingWithDeirdre.com.

Use this book for health-related content. The content of this book is for general instruction only. Each person's physical, emotional, and spiritual condition is unique. The instruction in this book is not intended to replace or interrupt the reader's relationship with a physician or other professional. Please consult your doctor for matters pertaining to your specific health and dietary needs.

US ISBN Number: 978-0692667170
European EAN Number: 0692667172
Library of Congress Control Number: 2016904558
Printed in the United States of America

Book interior design by Jean Boles
jean.bolesbooks@gmail.com

Book cover by Tehsin Gul
colorofparadise1983@gmail.com

DEDICATION

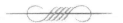

To my free-spirited daughter, who is a constant source of inspiration;

to my mother, who has always nurtured my inner voice;

to Jeff Wilder, for his patience and mentoring during all the years we've shared,

and to Edgis for sharing his teachings with me.

CONTENTS

ACKNOWLEDGEMENTS

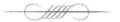

A Few Words Of Thanks

I am very grateful to my editor, Nancy K.S. Hochman, for her professional advice and guidance.

Much gratitude goes to Salomon Sanchez, whose compassion, humor, and assistance in every arena make so many things possible.

Special thanks to the Institute of Integrative Nutrition, the wonderful staff, colleagues and fellow alumni for all their insights, and their assistance with publishing this book.

Thank you, also, to my wonderful designers, who so artfully expressed my vision.

I also thank you, my readers, for your willingness to spend time with me in your search for natural, food-related solutions to good health. In the journey of life, we are all touched by personal health issues of one kind or another and are often challenged by the failing health of loved ones as they grow older.

In writing this book, my goal is to help you find clarity that leads to the journey back to perfect health for you and your loved ones. Knowledge is empowerment. It is also the key to avoiding many common health issues that are easily reversed in their early stages, when your body is communicating with you in the language of symptoms.

I wish you the benefits that come with understanding the deep connection between food and wellness. May this book assist you and your loved ones with avoiding much of the pain, anguish, anxiety and stress often caused by the challenges of less than optimum health.

May You Be Well Now and Enjoy Heath Every Day of Your Life.

News Flash:
When I announced that I was writing a book, everyone who knows me, and anyone who has tasted my food, or heard stories about my food, assumed that I was writing a cookbook.

I do indeed look forward to sharing my own recipes. Based on the Five Flavors of Chinese Medicine, these preparations are colorfully tantalizing to the eyes and delightful to the taste buds. Just as important, my unique cuisine, with its highest quality ingredients, is geared to optimizing health!

Before sharing my succulent, yet easy-to-prepare recipes with you, I very much want to help you acquire the foundation of delicious and healthful eating. This includes tips on the advantages and methods of easily growing your own fresh organic produce and herbs, or purchasing organic produce from local vendors. I provide you with information on identifying and selecting whole and minimally processed foods with which to line your pantry. I also include how to select and apportion higher nutrient snacks and sweets that will help satisfy your cravings without adding pounds to your waistline and stomach. I cover stocking your kitchen with safe and effective pots and pans, how to create alkaline water and prepare meals with it. Finally, I provide information on where to purchase these healthful products. It's not that this book is void of recipes either. I do touch on multiple preparations for these nutritious and delicious foods.

Reading this book, and following its suggestions, will help you benefit from significantly improved health, as it has many others whom I have coached, and who have written enthusiastic testimonials, included in this book. By the time you read my recipe book, tentatively titled, *Entertaining with Plates and Platters: "Beautiful and Delicious Meals in Minutes!* you'll already be enjoying the benefits of good health.

Meanwhile, please enjoy *Upgrade Your Life One Bite at a Time.*

If you want to have more energy and better health, try the recommendations set forth in this book for at least 30 days. And please share with me how things are working for you! Contact me via email: support@HealthyLivingWithDeirdre.com

Visit www.HealthyLivingWithDeirdre.com for your FREE companion guide that includes a shopping list and images of products! Also on my website is a marketplace where you can find all the products.

Note: If you are interested in a profitable and socially responsible business, utilizing my unique healing cuisine and Hospitality Real Estate experience, note that I'm seeking partners to launch a prepared foods company franchised restaurant brand and to establish a chain of eco-friendly life style hotels.
Contact me at:
support@HealthyLivingWithDeirdre.com

PROLOGUE

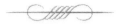

May I Introduce You To Some Of The Lives That I Have Touched?

Testimonials:

I spent five weeks living with Deirdre at The Harbor Rose. In that short amount of time, I learned much about healthy eating that has deeply impacted my life. I had been on oral diabetes medication for a few years. With the change to a plant-based diet, I was able to stop taking the medication and my blood sugar levels have stayed in the normal range for four years now. This is rare for someone in her 50s. I am thankful for what I have learned and am looking forward to learning more about healthful eating from Deidre's books!

– Susan Parks

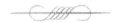

My name is J. Raphael. I'm 60 -years- old, and a frequent guest of The Harbor Rose. My eating patterns were influenced by Deirdre's healthy eating insights and unique and wonderful recipes. As a result of minor dietary changes, I found I was sleeping better than ever. I lost weight and gained the energy levels I enjoyed in my 30s. I have used Deirdre's insights for several years now, and I'm in better health now than ever before.

– J. Raphael, Visual Artist & Author; New York, New York

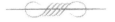

Last year, I turned 42 and had my third child. Deirdre, being a great friend, gave the best new baby gift ever: she fed me breakfast, lunch and dinner for a month. I regained my energy so much more quickly and recovered much faster than I had during my previous pregnancies. The food was simple, yet so yummy and combined in such interesting and exciting ways. My health and taste buds are better for it!

– Evelyn Melleby

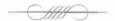

"If you really want to make a change, staying at The Harbor Rose B&B frequently and for a considerable amount of time will help you reap the rewards and benefits of a lifetime. You will find yourself asking questions that you never imagined!"
– Anonymous

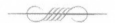

I have been working with Deirdre for two years now, and have learned so much about food and wellness. As a 43-year-old wife, and mother of three children, my household pantry has changed considerably, and my family has reaped the benefits of healthy living. Deirdre's guidance has significantly helped resolve my oldest daughter's menstrual issues, as she had been a junk food vegetarian. My 15-year-old daughter's severe acne problem is now resolved. Additionally, my 12-year-old son is no longer a borderline diabetic and his asthma is gone! My own health issues have also been resolved. I had severe pain in my breasts, dizzy spells, headaches, and joint pain, among other complaints. The doctors diagnosed me with cancer! After three months of eating only Deirdre's approved foods, utilizing her tips and recommendations on selecting and combining foods, and using her simple recipes, my symptoms disappeared. I credit my plant-based diet to these improvements; when I eliminated meat, my joint pain disappeared. Perhaps more important, when I was tested again, the doctors were unable to find the cancer that had previously shown up! An extra bonus is that we have all lost weight; I've lost three dress sizes. We've even begun to influence others: my daughter's soccer team prefers to eat soup and pasta at my place rather than going to the local pizzeria after the game. Additionally, extended family members are noticing the difference and a chain reaction is under way, as I am getting more questions about healthy eating patterns and requests for recipes. It has been an amazing journey to wellness. I am so grateful for the knowledge that Deidre has shared!

– Vilma Vasquez, Hospitality Food Service Professional

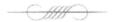

"When I first met Deirdre, I was twenty-six-years old. I was raised by my father, who was a physician. He led me to believe that the only answers to health and vitality come from the standard Western style of medicine. Deirdre allowed me to see a different way of finding solutions than the use of traditional Western medicine alone. Deirdre's solutions positively affected both my quality of life and health. She helped set me on a path that motivated me to move further and further into the holistic health and wellness lifestyle. I truly thank her for bringing awareness about the positive benefits of healthy and natural living. Today, at thirty-two, my body and mind are far more balanced than that of the twenty-six-year old that Deirdre first met. I remain always grateful for her inspiration!

– Patty

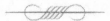

As I grew older, I started learning that food we eat plays a vital part in our health and well-being. I had been reading a lot on this subject, and tried to implement new and healthy eating habits into my diet. I either felt completely deprived or no different than before I made the change. It wasn't until I met Deirdre, at age 23, that I was able to be consistent with my diet. She introduced me to a new way of eating through her amazing recipes. They were not only delicious and satisfying, but also had the power to restore me back to optimal health! I cannot say enough about how her food has helped me. To sum it up, empowered is how I feel now!

– Chelsey Kennedy 25-years-old and now off prescription medication

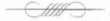

My name is Lani, and I am a 61-year-old woman who has struggled with the challenges of multiple sclerosis for close to 30 years. My thanks and praise go to Deirdre Ventura for her unwavering guidance and nutritional and spiritual support. She offered amazing insights into the direct correlation between nutrition and health. I am a testimony to the benefits of non-processed and organic foods that formed the core of my medical improvements. I made tremendous progress very quickly in improved balance, improved vision and overall strength and functioning. My dramatic improvement was evident to everyone, and I could only sing the praises of Deirdre's tips on healthy eating and simple recipes that gave me back my life. If you are a skeptic, try to be open-minded, and have faith in this amazing journey to health and wellness.

– Lani Roye LCSW

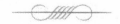

When I met Deirdre in 1988, I was 20 pounds overweight, and my skin color had an unhealthy reddish hue, due to the large quantities of red meat I was eating daily. Over a period of time, Deirdre convinced me that the way I was eating would continue to deteriorate my health: slowing down my metabolism, which would cause me to gain weight as I aged, and possibly impact my life span. As Deirdre changed my diet, I lost weight and gained a healthy look. I not only felt and looked better, I was able to function more effectively in my job as a supervisor. I am now 63 years old, and I have continued to follow the diet that Deirdre provided me over 28 years ago. I know if it were not for Deidre's recommendations, I would not have the great health that I have today.

– James Murphy

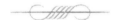

I have always been an athletic and active person. I have had the benefit of being healthy most of my life. When I was in college and working full time, I was surviving on fast food due to my limited budget. I began gaining weight, which caused me to feel less confident about my body image. I was also experiencing abdominal pain that on two occasions became so severe that I went to the hospital. My strategy was to exercise like crazy to restore my body.

Then, at the age of 25, I had the good fortune to arrive at The Harbor Rose. In getting to know Deirdre, I learned another way of life. Although I was aware that eating fruits and vegetables is important for good health. I did not like them, so I avoided them. I had a lot of resistance to changing my mentality!

Deirdre provided knowledge allowing me to change at a pace I was comfortable with, and I found support in making changes as I was struggling with my old habits.

Spending time at The Harbor Rose had a life changing impact on my life and my health. I was introduced to interesting versions of salads, soups and vegetables. Deirdre invited me to taste foods and I experienced many different flavors. Her foods are prepared in very different and colorful ways. Deirdre's unique and interesting cuisine changed my life; I began finding vegetables delicious! I learned how easy and affordable it can be to eat fruits and vegetables and live a healthier life. I've learned how to make better food choices and that excessive exercise was not the solution to the effects of a poor diet. I soon reduced my intestinal inflammation, restored my digestive tract, and learned the circumstances that caused the discomfort and pain in the first place! All of a sudden, it was no effort to enjoy good food and good health, while exercising less. I now have maintained a healthy weight, and experience more and longer lasting energy.

I am truly grateful for all I have learned and will continue to learn about food and health.

– Salomon Sanchez, age 27

INTRODUCTION

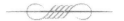

I've spent nearly 50 years exploring plant based foods and prepared food products. I have learned many short cuts to healthy eating habits. You, too, will learn how to spot high quality and low quality ingredients by ignoring the large print and trusting the logos of organic, fair trade and Non GMO products, to name a few. With this knowledge, you can also learn to reverse imbalances both **before** and **after** they begin to degrade your quality of life.

I have no affiliation, nor receive any benefit, from any of the products, companies or stores that I recommend in this book. My goal in recommending these products is simple and direct: I've successfully used these products and believe they are the best available at this time. Be aware that products can and do change; water quality and ingredient lists of supplements and prepared foods also change. Small artisan food companies are often bought by bigger companies who sometimes alter ingredients and or processing. So continue to check labels, even if you have always bought that product.

My first experience with an ingredient change was a painful one. As a kid, Ritz Crackers was a favorite. One day, after eating a handful of crackers, I had a terrible stomachache. What was my first instinct? I grabbed the box and looked at the ingredients. I discovered that the company had replaced butter with lard. I felt betrayed. As a vegetarian, this did not sit well with me one bit! As a kid I felt powerless, and was unable to express my frustration with Nabisco, who manufactures Ritz Crackers. Companies do change their high-cost ingredients to low-cost ingredients, suspecting that the customer will never know the difference

Needless to say, I never ate a Ritz Cracker again. Lesson learned: always check the ingredients before buying or consuming a food product.

The Benefits Of Smart Eating Habits

When you implement each upgrade for 30 days, replacing highly processed, unhealthful, and genetically engineered ingredients with fresh, rainbow-colored fruits and vegetables, and minimally processed foods, you will be amazed by the results! Many problems and annoying symptoms will simply disappear! The more upgrades you make, the better you will feel!

How does better health translate for you? Losing some weight? Clearer skin? Sleeping more deeply? Gaining weight? Thinking more clearly? Having more energy? Being allergy free?

You can restore your energy, your laughter, your vitality, and your quality of life by learning to ask the right questions and reading labels before purchasing and consuming food. As you restore your health, one bite at a time, you will find that a strong, healthy body hidden within will reveal itself before your very eyes.

As a sculptor says... *"I remove all that is not part of my masterpiece one stroke at a time with intention."*

By eliminating foods that rob you of your health, the true, healthful you will unfold!

I can provide you with pages of scientific facts and data culled from research over many years, and in some cases, I do. But that's not the purpose of this book. The purpose of this book is to provide a shortcut or "cheat sheet." You don't have to know everything. All you have to do is learn enough to make better choices, and then enjoy the results! Interested in learning more? I hope this book inspires you to delve further into more mindful eating patterns.

Follow the recommendations and enjoy delicious, satisfying, nutritious foods that provide healthy results nearly instantly.

How To Use This Book:

Taking into account your personal predilections, this book provides an introduction to healthy eating patterns, including the benefits of eating appetizing rainbow-colored foods, immune system building alkaline foods, whole organic foods and "taste bud tantalizing" freshly picked foods. Upgrade your condiments and utilize herbs and spices that promote healthy bodies while adding delicious flavors to your meals. Upgrade your palate and your plate from ordinary to extraordinary with color and powerful ingredients that enhance your immune system and strengthen your body. This book also addresses reasons for avoiding genetically engineered food, and ways to limit or exchange processed foods for better healthful alternatives. Additionally, it provides information on powerhouse nutrients, less damaging dairy food selections, and lists of substitute ingredients and alternative products and snack foods with higher quality ingredients that will keep your body trim and fit.

"You don't have to understand the sophisticated technology that makes a cell phone work to enjoy the benefits of having a cell phone!"

Don't worry. You don't have to learn to be a nutritionist, a research scientist or a chef to benefit. This simple and easy-to-read book removes all the guesswork, so you can enjoy your upgrades one bite at a time! Seeking a certain food? Look up the product in the book, replace it with a higher quality version, and feel the difference! Are you a person who writes lists? Cross reference your shopping list with this book and make upgrades each time an item appears.

Just a note: there are some whole foods that are not listed in this book largely because the food is uncommon or difficult to find. The foods that are included are high nutritional whole foods that represent all the colors found in the rainbow.

I have listed a few of my favorite foods in each category and hope you are inspired to explore and find many others that you will enjoy in years to come. I have also omitted prepared foods, spices and condiments that contain ingredients that rob you of your health and well-being. These include dyes and processed foods with additives and chemical ingredients. A good rule of thumb is to focus on consuming foods with ingredients that are recognizable in the produce aisle or in your Grandma's kitchen!

Are You Ready?

The foods we choose to eat are influenced by so many factors. Some people simply eat what is placed in front of them; others are more particular about the foods they consume. Some choose foods largely for enjoyment, others with health in mind. Some suffer from eating foods that "do not agree with them"; others freely eat, without complications, whatever they want. These differences also extend to food preparation: some people love dabbling in the kitchen; others choose to stay far away.

Our approach to food is a very personal choice. As our lives change, as we grow, develop, and mature, one thing remains constant. Change! The foods we eat also change, based on the neighborhood we live in, the seasons, availability, and the community we share. I invite you to set a goal for your health and well-being. It does not have to be a lofty goal, but rather small, achievable steps in the right direction. I encourage you to align the foods you consume with your personal goals for your health and well-being.

At a very young age, I knew I was a vegetarian living in a house of meat eaters. You may be the meat-eater living in a house of vegetarians! It does not really matter where you are on the spectrum. What matters is that you are taking healthful steps to arrive at where you want to be!

Contact me at www.healthLivingWithDeirdre.com or send me an email at support@HealthyLivingWithDeirdre.com. I'd love to hear about your journey.

My first self-healing journey restored my health solely by changing my diet. I found myself in a hospital bed as a young child, inflicted with agonizing stomach pains.

Once released from the hospital, I continued my trips from doctor to doctor and test to test. I was finally diagnosed with a bleeding duodenal ulcer. The doctors were baffled. The understanding at the time was that ulcers were adult disorders caused by stress. Although a precocious child, I was too young to effectively communicate my thoughts and feelings, but sensitive enough to allow what I learned to affect me physically. My upset began when I realized that my parents, people whom I loved, were feeding me my friends in the animal kingdom. To make things worse, my doctors prescribed the Standard American Diet, heavy in meat, dairy and processed foods, which neither agreed with my body, nor my spirit. I intuitively knew these foods were not for me.

After a clear nod to my mom that I was not going to eat the foods she set before me, that I had other foods in mind, my healing journey began. I eliminated meat, eggs, poultry, fish, seafood, cereal, processed foods wheat and dairy—with the exception of small amounts of high quality imported cheese. No more processed cheese food or instant potatoes for me!

I was finally enjoying real fermented foods, including pickles and sauerkraut, and whole fresh fruits and vegetables—mostly raw or slightly cooked, yet crunchy—and salads. I eliminated canned and boxed food and frozen food, except petite peas, which I loved. Within a few days my stomach pain subsided and my mom happily allowed me to continue designing my own diet.

CHAPTER ONE

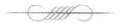

Let's Look At Your Body As A Business And Study The P & L Statement

I invite you to look at your body as a business Profit and Loss (P & L) statement. Just like a business has to be profitable, providing you with a high quality life, so must your diet.

The heart of every business is in the math. All businesses have expenses and receive revenue. The P & L lists all the revenue and the expenses of operating the business. If you sell an item for $10 and it costs $11 to produce the item, you are certainly not going to be in business very long!

By eating healthy foods, you are depositing "money": good health and well-being into your bank account. Conversely, by eating unhealthy foods, you are withdrawing from your health account.

Most successful companies invest in their future by allocating resources into research and product development. This provides longevity for the company and the opportunity to be on the cutting edge of new trends. When there is a proven system in place, you will miss neither an important observation, nor trend.

As You Select Your Food, Ask Yourself These Questions:

1. Am I doing research? If the answer is "yes," then you are keeping a food journal, noting your feelings, energy level, sleep, and excretion patterns. Just like a business person

conducting research and development, you are collecting data and enjoying a learning experience. Congratulations! At the same time, you're becoming a scientist!

Research and discovery are life-long processes! Our bodies and our lives are always changing, so the process is ongoing.

Remember to act like a scientist and invest in research and development for a healthy and profitable future!

2. How profitable is this product? What does your profit margin need to be in order to be successful? What type of profit margin do you need to maintain excellent health? If you are healthy and manage stress well, you are more likely to tolerate lower profit margins (and have more flexibility) when making food choices.

3. Is your company or body sick? Are the professionals recommending bankruptcy? Are you experiencing debilitating symptoms? This could be simple reoccurring aches and pains or an emotionally devastating illness that has now become part of your identity.

If the answer is yes to these questions, to stay in business—or to restore your health—it's time to execute the plan to restore profitability: your health and your quality of life.

This simple book will show you how to make better choices and upgrade your life and your health one bite at a time!

Perhaps you have no interest in business. The same concept applies to a savings account. We create savings accounts for all kinds of purposes, college funds and retirement, to name a few. We save for a large purchase like a house or a car and we utilize and benefit from investment accounts. The idea remains the same when we're talking about health. You make deposits with one action step.

Every time we put something in our mouth, it's an action step. Every time we open a package or select an item at the grocery store it's an action step. Each action step has the opportunity to be a withdrawal from your bank account of health or a deposit into your bank account of health. Whether those deposits are large or small, they require the same effort: moving the food from source to the plate to your mouth. The larger (higher quality) the deposit, the faster you reach your goal.

Healthy foods are "high profit" foods that equal large deposits. The more interest you earn in an account, the faster your account grows. By upgrading your food choices, you are not only making an investment in your health today, you will also enjoy the benefits in years to come. When you stay the course, your investments (your choices) will pay high dividends in the future!

The Benefits Of Buying Organic, Pesticide And GMO Free Foods

Somehow Deirdre takes vegetables that I hate and mixes them together into something that I love!

– Robbie Pellicane, age 13

Always Buy Organic!
There are countless reasons to buy organic.

First, let's explore the environmental reasons. Pesticides are designed to kill insects. However, in the larger scheme, insects are keeping us alive! Without the pollination of insects, we will not have plants that feed us. God intended us to co-exist in nature, but for generations we have spent our time controlling and manipulating nature.

Here's something else to consider: we use toxin-containing insecticides to kill insects that have a very short life span; the average lifespan for an ant is 40 – 60 days. Evolution assists every new generation in becoming stronger and more resistant to insecticides. Humans, who of course have a much longer life span, do not benefit from this evolutionary advantage that makes them far less resistant to toxins. The bottom line: insecticides make bugs stronger and humans sick and weak.

It's true that we are no longer farming with strong insecticides such as DDT, which was banned for agricultural use in the US in December of 1972. Yet, according to the FDA, traces of DDT have been found in the American food supply in recent years, despite its having been banned. Some 40 years later, it's affecting our food supply! The Center for Disease Control (CDC) conducted a test that found DDT breakdown product (DDE) in the blood of 99% of those subjects!

Girls exposed to DDT before puberty are five times more likely to develop breast cancer in middle age, according to the President's Cancer Panel. Studies show a range of human health effects linked to DDT and its breakdown product, DDE, including various cancers, low birth weights and miscarriages.

> For more information about the health risks of DDT exposure visit http://www.ncbi.nlm.nih.gov/pmc/articles/PMC2737010/

Additionally, studies from the United States and Sweden suggest that body burdens of DDT and/or DDE may be associated with the prevalence of diabetes.

The aforementioned are, unfortunately, only a few examples of the mounting evidence of environmental health hazards of our historical farming practices. Today's conventional farming practices are not necessarily all that much better.

In excess of 80,000 chemicals are now commercially available for use by agriculture and industry, and many potentially toxic compounds have been embraced to increase productivity and financial gain (Erickson 2009).

Both the number of toxicants in the environment and rates of toxin-related diseases have increased dramatically in the past 60 years, and countless published studies attest to a link between toxicants and health risks. For instance, comprehensive reviews highlight numerous studies that have identified a positive relationship between exposure to pesticides and the development of certain cancers, as well as adverse reproductive, metabolic and mental health effects (Sanborn et al. 2004, Maroni & Fait 1993).

In the 1990s researchers in the United States conducted a large prospective cohort study of pesticide applicators and their spouses, known as the Agricultural Health Study. The study identified links between various pesticides and prostate, lung, rectal and colon cancers (Alavanja et al. 2003, Alavanja et al. 2004, Lee et al. 2007).

Children are particularly vulnerable to the toxic effects of chemicals for a number of reasons: they exhibit more hand to mouth behavior; they eat and drink more per kilogram of bodyweight than adults; their skin is more permeable and their livers do not metabolize chemicals as efficiently (Sanborn et al. 2004).

Unlike industrially produced food, which makes generous use of pesticides, organic foods are full of minerals and other phytonutrients necessary for a healthy body and mind. Factory farming practices are all about large-scale production, food that looks perfect, ships well, has a long shelf life and is readily available through premature harvesting. This translates into less tasty produce, lacking in essential nutrients. Conventional farming practices are anything but about taste and nutritional value. Try a raw organic carrot and a conventional one side by side in your own taste test. I think you'll find the conventional one has little if any flavor, while the organic one is indeed tasty. Interestingly, sometimes organic carrots are even less expensive in the markets!

Organic Nutrient Rich Foods Are Less Expensive In The Long Term

Although you are perhaps paying more for organic foods at the point of purchase, when taking into account nutritional value, organic produce is actually less expensive! Organic fruits and vegetables provide you with far more nutrition and health benefits than factory farmed produce. You may also reduce costs of organic produce by joining a Community Supported Agriculture (CSA) organic farm. A CSA farm is a network or association of individuals who have pledged to support one or more local farms, with growers and consumers sharing the risks and benefits of food production. I have been a member of our local CSA for over 20 years and the produce is picked and on the table in the same day! And it's picked at the peak of perfection! An added bonus is it's educational for our children to learn about where our food comes from, and it's an added benefit to enjoy a personal connection with the farmer growing our food! By consuming more organic produce, I think you'll find that you'll experience fewer doctor visits and spend less money on supplements and drugs.

GMO...Avoiding The Dangers

Genetically modified foods, or genetically engineered foods (GMOs), are foods produced from organisms whose genetic material has been artificially manipulated in a laboratory. This relatively new science creates unstable combinations of plant, animal, bacterial and viral genes that do not occur in

A new study recently published in the *Journal of Organic Systems* last September examined US government databases. Researchers searched for GE (Genetically Engineered) crop data, to see if a correlation exists between GE crop data and 22 different diseases.

nature or through traditional crossbreeding methods. GMO foods have been known to cause systemic inflammation, the basic building blocks of disease.

The Top 10 prepared / processed foods that include GMO ingredients are baby formula, canned soups, frozen foods, milk, meat, soda, tofu, vegetable and canola oils, sweetened juices and cereal. Especially when it comes to these types of foods, look for the label: Non GMO or organic. Interestingly, 38 countries, including 28 nations in Europe, and Mexico, have banned GMO crops. If organic food is unavailable, it is better—from the "lesser of two evils perspective"—to chance eating foods with pesticides rather than those that are genetically modified. There are ways of detoxing your body of pesticides. When it comes to GMO foods, we may be unable to reverse the consequences.

One of the best studies ever done to document the dangers of GM foods found that overall, inflammation levels were a significantly 2.6 times higher in GE-fed pigs than those fed a non-GE diet, and male pigs fared worse than the females.

Here's a list of countries that banned genetically modified food.

A European Commission spokesman, Enrico Brivio, confirmed to Reuters that the 19 countries opting out are: Austria, Belgium for the Wallonia region, Britain for Scotland, Wales and Northern Ireland, Bulgaria, Croatia, Cyprus, Denmark, France, Germany, Greece, Hungary, Italy, Latvia, Lithuania, Luxembourg, Malta, the Netherlands, Poland and Slovenia.

United States: Only the California counties of Mendocino, Trinity and Marin have successfully banned GM crops. Voters in other California counties have tried to pass similar measures but failed.

Australia: Several Australian states had bans on GM crops but most of them have since lifted them. Only South Australia still has a ban on GM crops.

Japan: The Japanese people are staunchly opposed to genetically modified crops and *no GM seeds are planted in the country.* However, large quantities of canola oil are imported from Canada, which is one of the world's largest producers of GMO canola oil.

New Zealand: No GM foods are grown in the country.

Ireland: All GM crops were banned for cultivation in 2009, and there is a voluntary labeling system for foods containing GM foods to be identified as such.

Austria, Hungary, Greece, Bulgaria and Luxembourg: There are bans on the cultivation and sale of GMOs.

France: Monsanto's MON810 GM corn had been approved but its cultivation was forbidden in 2008. There is widespread public distrust of GMOs that has been successful in keeping GM crops out of the country.

Madeira: This small autonomous Portuguese island requested a countrywide ban on genetically modified crops last year and was permitted to do so by the EU.

Switzerland: The country banned all GM crops, animals, and plants on its fields and farms in a public referendum in 2005, now extended until 2017.

India: Recently, a committee of Supreme Court appointed experts have called on the Indian government to establish a 10-year ban on Monsanto's GMO crops, based on the growing resistance of GMO crops to herbicides, which has led to super weeds and super insects.

Thailand: The country is currently trying to embrace both sides—producing organic foods for some countries at a high price, while moving towards embracing more and more GM crops. This country has also tried declaring some areas GMO-free zones in order to encourage other countries to trust their foods.

There is no required GMO labeling of foods in the United States. This also includes GMO foods used as an ingredient or used as animal feed remain unlabeled. There are powerful companies working to deliver fresh, unlabeled GMO produce to our market shelves.

To stay up to date on GMO issues, visit www.nongmoproject.org.

CHAPTER TWO

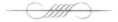

Business 101: Things You Need To Know About Foods That Efficiently Keep Your Motor Running

A Fresh Food Overview

The longer the shelf life, often the less profitable the nutrient value of the food. Let's return for a moment to the business metaphor. Business owners strive to represent high profit margin products or services in the local marketplace. This makes for a healthy business and a healthy body.

Did you know that not-from-concentrate orange juice can be stored for up to a year in million-gallon tanks before being bottled and sent to grocery stores? *Source: Investigation by Alissa Hamilton.*

Apples, when stored properly, can be up to a year old when they arrive at the grocery store. While these apples are safe to eat, fresh apples are best, another reason to buy fresh from an apple grower, or to consume apples in season. The same thing pertains to potatoes, which can be stored up to 11 months before arriving at your supermarket.

The shortest time between harvest and table equates to more life force = more nutrition = higher (health) profits. It's better for the environment and there are fewer opportunities for contamination. Eating local foods provides the opportunity to know our local farmer and be connected to our food supply and nature as we are enjoying and eating what's in season.

Locally grown, organic produce is the most desirable. Freshly picked produce is second best, and freshly store bought produce follows in line. If these are not options, then purchase food that is frozen or jarred. The trusty can is the least desirable choice for several reasons. First, cans are made from aluminum, which, some studies suggest, is related to the development of Alzheimer's disease. Second, cans are often lined with Bisphenol (BPA), which is a petroleum-based plastic. When cans are sealed they are heated and the contents is "cooked" providing the opportunity for

Processed foods and prepared foods are anything that is not a whole food. For example, a sardine with the head and eyes and all the bones intact, and with no oil or seasoning added, is a whole food. Clearly, there are different levels of processing. An apple is a whole food; applesauce and apple pie are processed or prepared foods. Moving down the line, an apple flavored pop tart is a highly processed item that contains a suggestion of apple. Mock Apple Pie, a recipe at one time found on the box of Ritz crackers, has no apples at all!

the aluminum and the BPA to leech into the food. Additionally, foods that are canned often don't meet the quality standards for freshness, reducing their nutritional value.

If you want processed food, either cooked or raw, it's generally best to "do it yourself." The first step in processing is washing; the second step is cutting; the third step is a choice—cook or eat raw—and the fourth step involves combining and seasoning. Let's keep it simple!

Why Is Freshly Picked So Important?

The fresher the food the more life force or profit it contains. If you can eat the fruit while it's still on the plant, while it's still connected to its source energy, then you have grabbed the brass ring! Enjoy as many raw foods as possible, as they provide enzymes for digestive health and improve waste elimination. It is preferable to eat raw foods before eating cooked foods when enjoying a meal, as the enzymes in raw food aid in the digestion of cooked foods.

Lettuce can be a few days old or up to two weeks old when it arrives on the grocery store shelves, depending on a variety of factors, including shipping distances and the type of lettuce.

Once A Foodie Always A Foodie!

There's nothing like freshly picked food, because of its super high profit. When we were kids, we'd jump in our little 16-foot boat with the 3-horse power engine and travel around the harbor to Cold Spring Harbor. We'd tie up the boat. With our camping equipment, we'd start the mile walk to the cornfields. We set up our camping equipment, and started the Sterno fire going to boil water. We would then dip the ripe corn directly into the pot. The corn would heat up and we would eat it right on the stalk. You have not really experienced fresh corn until you eat it this way! All the sugars turn to starch after the corn is picked and separated from its life source. The sweeter the corn, the less time has passed between picking and eating.

Always Question Advertisements

Many people acquire their nutritional information from advertising: Drink orange juice, which is rich in vitamin C. Yes, it is. However, vitamin C is lost due to oxidation as the juice is exposed to air. So make your own single servings or simply eat an orange!

Additional Information on Profit Foods and Food Types

The Benefits Of Alkalizing Food

It's simple. A fish cannot live in the desert sand and a cactus cannot live in the ocean.

The guidelines in the book outline the basics of simple daily choices to alkalize your systemic tissue, keeping your system profitable and healthy!

When your body PH is alkaline, inflammation and countless other pathogens and degenerative diseases cannot survive. The result is good health! Seeking long-term good health? Keep reading.

Alkalizing foods are defined by how the food affects the body system, not the intrinsic PH of the food. One might think that citrus is acidic, yet it is alkalizing to the body. Corn, wheat, meat, dairy and refined sugars are acid forming in the body.

Alkalizing vegetables include broccoli, carrots, cauliflower, celery, cucumber, garlic, lettuce, onions, parsley, peppers, seaweed, spinach, sweet potatoes and yams. Alkalizing fruits include apple, banana, berries, cantaloupe, rapes and raisins, melon, lemon, limes, tangerine, pineapple, raspberries, and watermelon.

And many spices are alkaline, including pink Himalayan salt!

Naturally, some foods are more alkalizing than others and charts vary a bit. However, the message remains the same: replace processed and refined foods with fresh ones and eat more of your favorite alkaline-producing foods.

Here are a few links to some food alkaline charts:

http://greenopedia.com/alkaline-acid-food-chart/

http://www.energiseforlife.com/acid-alkaline-food-chart-1.1.pdf

http://www.essense-of-life.com/topic_A-701/Alkaline+and+Acidic+Food+Chart+Health+Toxic.htm

A Definition Of Glycemic Load And Why It Matters Even If You're Not Diabetic!

The glycemic load (GL) of food is a number that estimates how much the food will raise a person's blood glucose level. Eat high profit low glycemic load foods. Low glycemic load foods are typically fresh, whole and unprocessed. The goal here is to eat and have energy for 3-4 hours without being hungry or feeling like the food is still being processed by your digestive track. Low glycemic foods maintain blood sugar levels. High glycemic foods, such as refined sugars and processed foods create blood sugar spikes. The body responds with insulin to restore balance. This cycle leads to inconsistent energy levels throughout the day. Low glycemic foods will allow you to enjoy long lasting, slow burning energy.

I was just giving my daughter a lesson on glycemic load. We built a fire from nice sturdy oak logs, which burn hot and long. (Slow burning food provides long lasting fuel.) Then we took some paper and threw it into the fire, resulting in quick flash flames. There was a moment of high heat... Quick as a flash, it was gone! The burning paper is a symbol for high glycemic load foods that we consume: we experience a quick burst of energy, and then "burn out." The energy created is comparable to energy received by very low profit foods—foods with high glycemic levels.

When you choose to eat high glycemic foods, such as pasta or bread, it's best to combine them with low glycemic load foods, such as tomatoes, salad greens and peas. Try balancing them with raw carrots, celery, spinach, mushrooms, or cooked broccoli and green beans, all of which have NO glycemic load! The

Are you in the mood for a pasta dinner? To balance your meal, start with salad and soup. The relationship of whole grain pasta to cooked vegetables should be one-third pasta to two-thirds cooked vegetables. Enjoy fruit or coconut ice cream for desert.

majority of the meal should consist of low glycemic foods, in order to make the meal more profitable for your health.

And Then There Was Soy—Touted As The Vegan Miracle Protein!

In 3,000 BC, ancient writing suggested that the Chinese recognized the unfitness of soybeans for human consumption in their natural form. Now 5000 years later, we are once again beginning to understand ancient wisdom.

Many early studies indicated that soy was a healthful food. If you examine the science, and more recent studies, you will find that thousands of studies link soy to malnutrition, digestive distress, immune system breakdown, thyroid dysfunction, cognitive decline, reproductive disorders and infertility—even cancer and heart disease.

Soy contains several damaging compounds, including phyto-estrogens / isoflavones which mimic human estrogen, can block normal estrogen and disrupt endocrine function, cause infertility, and increase your risk for breast cancer.

There are also additional concerns. Soy contains goitrogens, an agent that blocks the synthesis of thyroid hormones and can cause hypothyroidism and thyroid cancer. In infants, consumption of soy formula has been linked with autoimmune thyroid disease. This compound also interferes with iodine metabolism. Soy is also high in phytic acid (phytates).This compound reduces assimilation of calcium, magnesium, copper, iron and zinc, and contains high levels of aluminum, which are toxic to your nervous system and kidneys.

Have you ever wondered why soy milk often has added synthetic (toxic) vitamin D2? It's because soy foods increase your body's vitamin D requirement. Soy foods also contribute to B12 deficiency, as they contain a compound that is similar to B12 that cannot be utilized by the body.

Additionally, glyphosate (also called Round Up), an herbicide used for soy crops, was identified by a French team of researchers and found to be carcinogenic.

And let us not forget that 90% of soy in the US is genetically modified (GMO) and 78% of the soy worldwide is GMO.

MSG is often added to improve the taste and often appears on the ingredient list as "spices."

For all the reasons above, I strongly recommend eliminating or limiting your soy intake if the soy product is not fermented. Soy-based foods include tofu and Yuba (also known as bean curd), texturized vegetable protein (TVP), edamame (soybeans in their pods), Yakidofu, hydrolyzed vegetable (or plant) protein, Kinnoko flour, Natto, Kyodofu (freeze-dried tofu) Shoyu sauce and Terrikyaki sauce. Additionally, ingredients such as "natural flavor," "vegetable broth," vegetable starch," and "vegetable gum," may contain soy. There are many additional soy-based foods that have the word "soy" in them.

For more information and links to additional studies, visit the Westin A. Price Organization at: http://www.westonaprice. org/soy-alert/

One of them, soy lecithin, is often used to sweeten processed foods. In a study published in *Food and Chemical Toxicology*, the researchers concluded that soy lecithin was also found to be strongly estrogenic, a compound shown to disrupt thyroid and endocrine hormone production.

In 1985, researchers performed a study on rats to test the negative effects of soy lecithin intake during gestation. The researchers fed pregnant and newborn rats either a 2% or 5% soy lecithin preparation diet. The researchers concluded, "The results indicate that dietary soy lecithin preparation enrichment during development leads to behavioral and neurochemical abnormalities in the exposed offspring."

The Positive Side Of Soy—Fermented Soy

During the Ming dynasty, fermented soy appeared in the Chinese *Materia Medica* as a nutritionally important food and an effective remedy for diseases.

Even with fermented soy foods, a little is just enough. The nutrients found in miso, tempeh, and natto, consumed in the typical Asian diet, can be beneficial in small amounts—approximately one ounce a day—but can be harmful in higher amounts.

Miso, a fermented form of soy served as soup, has been regarded as a cure for radiation exposure and prevention.

In 1985 medical doctors Lidia Yamchuk and Hanif Shaimardanov, organized Longevity, the first macrobiotic association in the Soviet Union. At their hospital, they began incorporating miso soup into the diets of patients suffering from radiation symptoms and cancer, as well as acupuncture to treat many patients, especially those suffering from leukemia, lymphoma and other disorders associated with exposure to nuclear radiation. "Miso is helping some of our patients with terminal cancer to survive," Yamchuk and Shaimardanov reported. "Their blood (and blood analysis) became better after they began to use miso in their daily food."

Source: *Journal of Toxicological Pathology:* "Beneficial Biological Effects of Miso with Reference to Radiation Injury, Cancer and Hypertension.

Science has concluded that the longer the fermentation process, the greater the benefits to the test subjects.

How to buy freeze-dried organic miso powder

As always, it is important to be connected to our food sources, know our farmers whenever possible, and understand the quality standards and procedures our suppliers use to process, ship, handle and store the foods that we consume.

Note: A good source of high quality miso can be purchased through the website: www.NaturalNews.com.

Traditional fermentation destroys these anti-nutrients and is the only process that allows your body to enjoy soy's nutritional benefits.

CHAPTER THREE

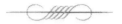

Let's Explore Dairy ... An Industry Powerhouse Of Influence

> An astounding 163 billion pounds of milk and milk products a year are produced by US dairy farmers!
>
> Statisa.com—The Statistics Portal

The US Dairy Annual Advertising Budget is $180 Million and the US government spends $30 billion annually in subsidies for animal products such as dairy. That's a total of $30,180,000,000 a year!

The Advertising is paying off, as the average American consumes over 600 lbs. of dairy products a year!

In 2007, the average American consumed 253.8 lbs. of milk a year in contrast to the average Mexican, who consumed less than half that amount at 115.18 lbs., the average Spaniard, who consumed 117 lbs. and the average Moroccan, who only consumed 50 lbs.

Clearly, cultural and business factors affect people's preference for and consumption of animal milk and animal milk products. Personally speaking, I went from mother's milk to table food. My mother reminds me that she tried to give me cow's milk in a bottle, but I consistently tossed the bottle across the room. Something inherently deep inside me made me realize that, at least for me, consuming another species' milk was very unappealing!

More recently, data has shown that cow's milk is far less than ideal for human consumption. It is important to recognize that milk is species specific. Cow's milk is designed for the baby cow to grow to 1,500 pounds into adulthood. A brief note about a humanist objection to cow's milk: mother cows produce not only the right type of milk, but also the right amount of milk for their calves. Drinking milk from cows one raises may rob the calf of sufficient nutrients.

There are also biological objections to drinking cow milk. Many people can't tolerate the antibiotics and growth hormones found in cow milk. The protein in cow milk is also hard to assimilate. That said, if you are hooked on drinking milk, I would recommend trying goat milk for starters. Proteins in goat milk are much smaller and easier for humans to digest than those in cow milk.

The ability to digest animal milk is also genetically based. Given that historically, Asians did not consume dairy, people of pure Asian descent may likely lack the required digestive enzymes to properly digest dairy. For these populations, and individuals who have trouble digesting milk, or who are lactose intolerant, I believe the best option is to consider the discomfort you may be experiencing and abstain from drinking milk, rather than taking pills that mask the discomfort.

Many studies have linked dairy consumption to respiratory issues, general congestion, and excess mucus production, constipation, and skin and digestive problems to name a few less severe side effects of dairy consumption. These are early warning signs not to be ignored. This is your system communicating with you. How are you responding?

For those who choose to drink cow milk, the best option is fresh raw milk—which is the most wholesome milk bought from the Amish farmer—or purchasing organic pasteurized milk that is antibiotic and growth hormone free. Fresh, raw milk is the most wholesome milk. Also, when I refer to the Amish farmer, it's a food source grown or raised by the Amish community.

Many people have asked me, "As a vegetarian, how are you sure you get enough protein?" Remember, animals and people in many communities worldwide derive their protein primarily from plants! There are many plants that provide protein, among them, beans, grains and even many vegetables. Industry uses scientific discoveries, such as the discovery of protein, to sell products, using advertising and often misleading information or half-truths! Don't be fooled.

Let's Explore Cheese And Yogurt

Things To Remember About Rennet

Cheese is acidic rather than alkaline, so we have to consume very small amounts and balance our cheese with high alkaline foods. I like to say, "Eat no more than three tablespoons of cheese a day in the winter and less in the other seasons." We are talking about real cheese, not processed cheese food. Hard cheese is more nutritious / higher profit than soft cheeses. A kosher seal on the label may indicate a higher quality, since non-animal rennet was used, but it also may be GMO. Rennet is the enzyme used to activate the milk to curdle into a cheese. Note that some soft cheeses, including ricotta and mascarpone, are made without rennet.

Below is a summary of the different kinds of rennet. Keep in mind that companies are not legally bound to disclose the type of rennet used on the label, so at times one just doesn't know what type of rennet a company is using. Again, it's best to buy organic, since all organic cheeses are made with the Non-GMO rennet.

1. Animal rennet (most expensive, up to twice the cost of alternatives)

2. Microbial rennet (mold derived rennet, harder to find, now often replaced by FPC GMO rennet) What is FPC you ask? In the late 1980s, scientists figured out how to transfer a single gene from bovine cells that codes for chymosin into microbes, giving microbes the ability to produce chymosin. These genetically modified microbes are allowed to multiply and cultivate in a fermentation process while they produce and release chymosin into the culture liquid. The chymosin can then be separated and purified. Chymosin produced using this method is termed fermentation-produced chymosin, or FPC.

Source: *Genetic Literacy Project May 15 the 2015 author Jon Entine & XiaoZhi Lim)*

3. FPC-Fermentation Produced Chymosin rennet (GMO)

4. Vegetable rennet (hard to source)

5. Citric acid or vinegar (often sourced from GMO corn)

Sadly, GMO is finding its way into our food supply in so many ways. Cheese is no exception.

How To Make The Best Selection If You Are Not Buying Organic And Can't Ask The Cheese Maker:

It's best to buy cheese not made in the US, but rather made in Europe, since GMO animal feed is not gown in Europe. That said, European countries do import 30% or so of their animal feed, which is often GMO and may contain GMO rennet.

Unfortunately, FPC (the process used to make rennet) has proven exempt from labeling requirements. Whether from European or American sources, EU and FDA regulations are vague when referencing ingredients that are considered trace. Some countries, such as France and Austria, are stricter with their labeling and exclusion of GMO foods. French and Austrian cheeses are likely safer than cheeses imported from other countries when it comes to GMO ingredients.

Additionally, sheep and goats can't tolerate growth hormones and antibiotics, so these are safer selections. If making a selection from only US made cheese, look for rBST Free (rBST is a growth hormone) Also, look for cheeses labeled Non GMO and grass fed.

To avoid all traces of GMO ingredients one must buy organic or know your farmer and cheese maker.

The local Amish farmer is again a great source for high quality cheese.

Some of the tastiest non-organic cheeses I've found include:

Authentic Greek Feta:	This cheese is packed in brine and made from sheep's milk. It's creamy, not too salty, and has a long shelf life. It's made with microbial rennet. We use it to make traditional Greek salads with tomatoes, cucumbers, Kalamata olives, red onion and an assortment of oregano from our "Plant and Pray Garden." A bit of lemon juice, olive oil and fresh ground rainbow pepper—it's a winning salad!
	Available: Trader Joe's

Pecorino Romano Grated Cheese:

This grated cheese is also made from sheep's milk. We use it very sparingly because it contains animal rennet. We do occasionally sprinkle it on soups, salads, and pizza. If you are a grated cheese fan, this may be an upgrade from many of the more common commercial brands.

It is available at Trader Joe's and has a blue plastic seal-wrap on the top.

Goat Cheese:

Goat cheese can often have a bitter aftertaste; making a selection can be a bit can be tricky. My favorite brand is Silver Goat Chevre Goat Cheese, made in the traditional European style. It is very creamy and sweeter than other brands and is made with microbial rennet.

Available: Trader Joe's

Cheddar:

English Ale Cheddar Cheese with Mustard is made with microbial rennet. I like to slice it very thin and place it between two apple slices. This works nicely as a snack or an addition to a tray of hors d' oeuvres.

Available: Trader Joe's

Organic Mozzarella:

Mozzarella is a standard if you love Italian food. I prefer brands that taste good in a fresh basil and tomato salad and that also melts well when baked. When making a salad I have a large bed of basil, large thick slices of tomatoes and a tiny bit of cheese to balance the alkalinity of the dish as best I can. I do the same thing when making pizza, using a suggestion of cheese—as little as possible. My favorite brand is Eco Meals Organic Amish Country Farmer. It's organic and made by small family Amish farmers, so it's also antibiotic and hormone free, not to mention, delicious.

Available: Whole Foods

Cambozola:

This is a triple cream soft rind blue cheese. I like to use this cheese to stuff celery stalks. Then I cut the celery into bite-size pieces. It's a nice addition to a platter when entertaining or can be enjoyed as a snack. As with any soft cheese, the flavors are richer when served at room temperature. My favorite brand is Trader Joe's, made in Germany. It's rBST free and made with microbial rennet.

Available: Trader Joe's

Sliced Chesses: If you are a fan of sliced cheeses, Applegate farms are the answer. They offer a wide variety.

Available: Whole Foods

When It Comes To Yogurt

When you consume a product, I believe it's important to know how the product is made and even how the product has traditionally been made, say 100 years ago. An Ikea pressboard piece of furniture and a piece of furniture that was carved from one piece of wood are hardly the same products; one is slapped together in a factory and the other is a craftsman's work of art. It is important to value and appreciate the work of a craftsman and upgrade your pallet. You can do so by actively involving yourself in making that product, or considering the homespun yogurt-making process.

Let's look at the how to make your first batch of homemade yogurt. First, we need animal milk and a starter culture. Where does the starter culture come from? There are a few places in nature to get the yogurt bacteria to make a starter culture. The most common are ant eggs or the soil around the entrance of an ant hill home. First collect some milk, then some ant soil or egg. Place the eggs or ant soil in sterile cheesecloth so it does not freely mix with the milk. Then follow the instruction on your yogurt maker. It is important to maintain temperature when making yogurt and a yogurt maker will help with this. In five hours or so the milk will set and will have the consistency of a gel. After the milk has set the gel is then strained to be sure there are no ant egg or soil residues. This will be the mother culture you use in the yogurt maker. Each time you make a generation of yogurt, you are also creating another mother culture. Most often, it's not until the fifth generation of yogurt or the fifth batch you make that you will experience consistent flavor from the mother culture. If you had to work this hard, how much yogurt would you consume?

Today's commercial mass-market yogurt producers often add sugar. Many companies add other sweeteners and some unrecognizable ingredients. This is especially true in those yogurt products being marketed to children. Again, if your child has respiratory issues, congestion, a running nose and slow bowel movements, or constipation, much of this will disappear when dairy is removed from the diet. My daughter loves yogurt, but because of the aforementioned factors, I limit both the number of servings and only give my daughter yogurt in the winter.

Yogurt is best consumed in the winter months for a reason. From a naturalist perspective, the calf is being weened in the summer / fall, so this is when the extra milk is available and it takes time to make yogurt in the traditional way. Many of the popular "yogurt" brands that you see advertised are not the real deal. The beneficial microbes are added to the dairy product just before the lid goes on in the assembly line, which does not guarantee that the probiotics are actually alive at the time you eat the product.

When making a selection, it is best, as previously mentioned, to select organic goat milk yogurt rather than cow milk yogurt. It's also best to select plain and add your own fruit or high quality sweeteners.

When eating yogurt, we make sure to have high alkaline vegetables in the same meal to balance the alkalinity of the meal, as dairy is very acidic. Besides, one cup of yogurt is a lot of dairy!

At the Harbor Rose B&B, we serve organic Redwood Hill Farm yogurt, which is kosher, and has no added low quality sugars. The vanilla-flavored yogurt has a bit of a maple syrup taste. Some of the other flavors use honey or apple juice to add a bit of sweetness. Many of our guests are pleasantly surprised at how tasty it is, and the smaller proteins are much easier to digest. If you are fond of the creamy single serve ritual of yogurt, try So Delicious brand coconut yogurt, an excellent nondairy alternative, although it does contains sugar.

The Many Ways Dairy Is Hidden In Processed Foods

Many processed foods have "hidden dairy," dairy that, due to wording, may not be recognized as such. If you are sensitive to dairy products, be forewarned, different wordings the dairy industry uses that you—as in processed foods—as a consumer may be unaware of include:

Acidophilus Milk

Ammonium (Calcium Caseinate)

Butter Solids

Buttermilk

Buttermilk Powder

Calcium Caseinate

Casein

Cream

Curds

Custard

Delactosed Whey

Demineralized Whey

Goat Cheese

Half & Half

Hydrolyzed Casein

Hydrolyzed Milk Protein

Hydrolysate

(Whipped Topping)

Iron Caseinate

Lactalbumin

Lactoferrin

Lactoglobulin

Lactose

Lactulose

Low-Fat Milk

Magnesium (Sodium Caseinate) Derivative

Natural Butter Flavor

Nougat

Paneer

(Potassium Caseinate)

Pudding

Recaldent

Rennet Casein

Sodium Solids

Sweetened Condensed

Whey Powder

Whey Protein Concentrate

Zinc Caseinate

I'm inviting you to be focused on the health of your body and your profits!

Let's Explore a Bit More About this Protein "Casein"

Casein is a protein found in mammal milk. There are two types of protein found in dairy products: casein and whey protein. Thirty-eight percent of the solid matter in milk is made of protein. Of that total protein, 80 % is casein and 20 % is whey. Cheese is made mostly of casein.

Casein's slow digestion rate puts great strain on the digestive system, according to Dr. Frank Lipman (an Integrative and Functional Medical expert). Dr. Neal Barnard, M.D. (founder of the Physician's Committee for

Casein is used in food for its scientific properties to thicken and congeal foods and possibly for its addictive properties to sell more products.

Responsible Medicine, a.k.a PCRM) found that in various studies, when dairy products were removed from the diet, cheese was the hardest food for people to give up. Dr. Barnard credits this finding to cheese being the most concentrated source of casein of all dairy products. PCRM also discovered that milk actually contains morphine, which can clearly be seen when milk is inspected under a microscope. Morphine is not added to cow's milk; cows actually produce these opiate-like chemicals on their own.

CHAPTER FOUR

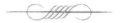

The Side Effect Of Perfect Health Is Perfect Weight!

The 80/20 Rule: *If you don't like what you see ahead... you're probably heading in the wrong direction....* Change your course just one degree and find yourself in a very different place in the years to come.

The **Pareto principle** (also known as the **80–20 rule**, the **law of the vital few**, and the **principle of factor sparsity**) states that, for many events, roughly 80% of the effects come from 20% of the causes

In business the 80/20 rule is 80% of your profit comes from 20% of your customers.

The 80/20 Goal For Health:
80% of your food is high profit fresh organic and 20% is research!

Assuming you are in reasonably good health, it's important to remember not to stress yourself out over trying to do "everything right." We are social beings, especially when it comes to food; it is okay to make choices that are not the best or ideal at time. It's more about being "aware" that you are making a less than desirable choice, about making decisions that consciously create a balance that works best for you.

Proper Food Combining: Fresh, Seasonal Foods Are Key Ingredients For Good Nutrition.

Food Combinations are Key

Grains + Vegetables or Fruit = Happy, Healthy, Profitable Body

Meat or Dairy or Nuts + Vegetables or Fruit = Happy Healthy Profitable Body

In short, eat proteins with vegetables, legumes or fruit. Proteins include any animal products such as chicken, fish, meat or dairy, seeds, nuts and beans. Avoid combining proteins with grains, as this interferes with absorption.

High quality and profitable whole grains include red and black rice, barley, quinoa, steel cut oatmeal and millet. Low quality forms of grains include anything made with flour or pressed out of an excursion machine. An example of the result of an excursion machine is often boxed cereals that feature consistent shapes, such as "o's" and "flakes." Other low quality grains include instant oatmeal, and wheat, white rice and brown rice, the latter of which, although better than white rice, provides far fewer nutrients than darker types of rice, such as mahogany and black rice.

Why Is Eating Local Food Combinations Important?

Nature has a unique way of balancing locally. For every local problem, there is a local custom or solution. It is wise to pay attention to cultural customs and eating patterns, because there is often an underlying health reason for them. For example, in Japan people consume large amounts of Sushi. Interestingly, there are several components to this unique cuisine and many practical health benefits. White rice is used; however, the seaweed balances this dish by adding high quality replacement minerals that were removed when the rice was processed. Additionally, the Wasabi mustard (the green lump served on the side) is a natural parasite remedy. Many larger fish, such as tuna, collect both parasites and heavy metals during their life in the ocean. The Wasabi neutralizes those parasites. The Black Tea the Japanese frequently drink bonds with the heavy metals so that their bodies excretes them rather than storing them in fat tissue. Consuming local indigenous foods ensures you are eating freshly picked produce, teeming with nutrients. It connects you to your local ecosystem. It also affords you the opportunity to enjoy different varieties that may not ship or store well and are therefore not commercially available.

Limit These Foods To Ensure Good Health And Control Weight

Your digestive track is 80% of your immune system. Caring for your digestive system and immune system certainly contributes largely to your goods health. A person with a "beer belly" or a lower tummy pouch is likely a victim of the Standard American Diet, the acronym for which is justifiably "SAD." The brown white and tan colors of meat, fish, dairy, bread, pasta, white rice and Idaho potatoes, along with low quality oils and lots of sugar and salt signal that they are loss leaders, lacking profit for you, the consumer, and yielding undesirable results. These foods are largely about making money for the companies that introduce these products into the food supply. They are of little or no nutritional value, and have little or no flavor without the added sugars and salts. The highly processed foods, coupled with clever advertising, are sometimes designed to trigger dopamine, an organic chemical that, amongst other factors, helps control the brain's reward and pleasure centers. These foods are often addictive, creating cravings and causing people to seek larger and more frequent helpings. This overworks the digestive track because the body is seeking nutrition, activating the survival mode that tells it "eat more!" Overweight people are often starving, nutritionally speaking.

If you are constipated, you have likely consumed too much "SAD' foods, such as GMO wheat, dairy, animal proteins and sugars. To reverse, eat three tablespoons of E3 Live, a frozen algae product found in Whole Foods, and a bunch of fiber fruits like figs and pineapple to resolve.

When To Eat?

Did you know that Japanese sumo wrestlers dedicate themselves to gaining weight? They largely accomplish their weight gain by eating meals after 9:00 pm and throughout the night. If you're looking to gain weight, follow the sumo wrestlers' example. If not, try avoiding eating later than 6:00 or 7:00 in the evening. Be sure to go to sleep only after digestion has been completed. Digestion requires two hours for a vegetarian meal, 3 hours if eggs, meat, fish or poultry are on the menu) When the body is sleeping, it's time for repair and other necessary body maintenance functions. It's best to not add digesting a meal to the time scheduled for repairs and maintenance!

The Higher the Nutritional Content the Less Food You Desire to Eat ...
High Quality = Less Volume = More Profit
More Profit & More Savings = Better Health

Juicers And Juicing

If you are looking to detox and lose weight safely and quickly, a juice fast may be just what the doctor ordered. Although I do not recommend juicing as a lifestyle choice, it can be very helpful at certain points in one's journey back to health. If you are suffering from any disease that is caused by inflammation, give juicing a try for, say, 7 – 10 days or more. This is a fresh juice only protocol, often called a juice fast. If you are on medication, be sure to work closely with your doctor to be sure you are being safely monitored, and be prepared to be amazed by the results.

Here is the reason that I don't recommend juicing as a lifestyle. If you are already in perfect health and you are consuming organic high nutritional content foods, it's better to chew your foods, the first step in digestion, rather than consuming them as juice. Chewing your food prepares your digestive track to properly receive the benefits of the food.

Although you can't chew freshly made juice in the same sense that you chew solid food, hold the juice in your mouth to activate saliva, and try to "chew" the juice with your teeth, as if it were a solid food. To learn more about the importance of chewing and other important healthy eating habits you may want to read *Power Eating Program: You are How You Eat*, by Lino Stanchich.

Some Of My Favorite Juicing Recipes:
Among my favorite juicing recipes, here is a family meal replacement Detox Recipe with plenty of herbs, and it is quite yummy!

The Herb Blend:

2 cloves garlic	2 medium-sized tomatoes
4 rainbow chard leaves and stalks	1 Bosc pear
6 - 8 celery stalks	1 lemon
½ bunch parsley	1 bunch watercress
½ bunch cilantro	1 English cucumber
1 bunch basil	1 bag of spinach
1 head romaine lettuce	4 carrots
4 stalks scallions	1 daikon radish

Once washed and juiced, add 1/2 tablespoon olive oil and 5 drops oil of oregano. Consume as a meal replacement, and remember to chew the liquids as long as you can before swallowing!

Variations on the Herb Blend Juice

4 rainbow carrots

1 head of red leaf lettuce

1 head of bok choy

4 tomatoes or a box of grape tomatoes

1 fresh fennel bulb, including the soft greenery

1 clove garlic

1 English cucumber

1 bunch parsley

1 bunch baby spinach

6 stalks of celery

1/2 bunch mustard greens

(See Herb Blend juice directions on previous page.)

Here's a Fruit Smoothie to enjoy:

1 pack frozen Acai

1 cup frozen organic strawberries

1 cup frozen organic wild blueberries

1 organic banana

3 ounces of hot green tea

Serve with mint from your Plant and Pray Garden

Liver Detox Juice – How to Improve your Complexion

Red Beets (start with 1 small beet per serving)

Garlic – small clove to taste

Olive oil

Oil of Oregano – a few drops to taste

On an empty stomach, try 2 to 3 ounces of the juice or one small red beet. Each day you can increase the amount, until you can comfortably consume a 16-ounce glass of red beet juice in less than 45 minutes. Be prepared, as this is a strong liver detox, so sip slowly, and if you feel lightheaded or dizzy, quickly drink 16 ounces or more of alkaline water. This will stabilize your

> **Note:** Detoxing and cleaning your intestines will also foster painless wet bowel movements.

system and lead the toxins to your urinary track more quickly. Also, remember that when you eat red beets, your urine will turn pink and your stool may be dark red. This is normal.

What You Need To Know When Selecting A Juicer:

There are four basic kinds of juicers:

(1) The first is the old-fashioned squeeze juicer or press that is hand operated. You might remember the old ones your grandmother may have used; they were often made of glass with a little ridge to catch the pits. I have one of these and use it every day for lemons and limes.

(2) The second kind is a centrifugal force design, which is typically less expensive and not as efficient as a masticating type.

(3) The third kind is an auger juicer, which operates at lower speeds and works well with soft items, such as greens. However, it does not succeed as well in juicing hard items such as beets and carrots.

(4) The fourth type is the masticating juicer. Masticating means to chew, to grind or knead into a pulp. Masticating juicers use high-speed rotation and "cutting teeth" to grind or chew. The downside to this type of juicer is that small amounts of the pulp or fiber may be separated and discarded or used for compost.

I have a commercial grade Champion Juicer. It is the masticating type—really old, powerful and easy to clean. In the more than 20 years that I've had this juicer, I have never had to replace any parts. Replacement parts are, nonetheless, available. If you're looking for a juicer or replacement parts already used, they're easily found on Craig's List. You can still find new Champion Juicers; best of all, they come with a 10-year limited warranty

Other more modern versions that appear to hold up include the Vitamix juicer. The benefit of this juicer is that all the material is turned into juice; there is nothing for the composter, so you are enjoying the benefits of the fiber in the juiced foods.

When selecting a juicer, remember to be sure that the parts that come into contact with the food are not made of aluminum!

There are so many juicers on the market, do the research to be sure you are making the best selection for you.

Note: Many juicers come with recipes for juicing—have fun exploring!

Let's Decode The Ingredients List In Prepared Foods And Beverages

Discover Added Sugars… And Vote "No" With Your Dollars!
The United States Department of Agriculture (USDA) reports that the average American consumes anywhere between **150** to **170 pounds** of refined sugars in one year! You may be thinking, "I do not consume that much." You very well may be, if you are not reading labels.

It is imperative that you read the ingredients, not just the nutritional grid. Ingredients are listed in descending order by weight. For example, if you are buying what you think is juice and sugar is the first ingredient, water the second, and juice, the third ingredient, the product has more sugar than juice by weight. Sugar in all its forms is a very cheap ingredient. If a company wants to increase profits and lower food costs, adding sugar is a popular way to accomplish these goals! The best choice is to make your own juice by slowly chewing many varied fresh fruits and vegetables. Next best is using a juicer or purchasing freshly made juice at a juice bar. When I enjoy juice, I want pure juice, without unnecessary ingredients that provide empty calories that make withdrawals from your bank account of health. For the sake of your weight and health, you might want to consider the same.

Discover Added Sugars and Vote "No" with Your Dollars!

Vote with Your Dollars as if Your Life Depends on it!

Consumers' consistent shopping patterns communicate the most powerful messages with each transaction. The choices made by the collective effects all, both today and for generations to come!

According to the Nonprofit Food Label Movement, there are almost 100 different names for sugar and sugar alcohols on ingredient lists. Ideally, don't purchase products with added sugar. And remember, the FDA is always approving more words for sugar. There are many ways that sugar can be hidden in the ingredient list. Learn to recognize sugar content by reviewing this list of different sugar forms.

Food additives have entered our food supply relatively recently— in the last generation. It was not until 1958 that the Food and Drug Administration (FDA) enacted the Food Additives Amendment, requiring manufacturers of new food additives to establish safety. The FDA publishes in the Federal Register the first list of substances generally recognized as safe (GRAS). The list contains nearly 200 substances in 1958 and has grown to over 10,000 in less than 60 years. Although the FDA recognizes these additives as safe, don't be fooled.

The human body has two responses to substances that we ingest. The body recognizes one substance as food, slowly breaks the food down, absorbs the nutrients and creates energy that fuels the body. Likewise, the body does not recognize nonfood substances, such as additives and preservatives, as food. Remember, preservatives are geared toward preserving food from breaking down or being digested by bacteria and enzymes. The body responds by storing these nonfoods as fat. When considering health and wellness, this is essential information!

Did you ever notice the heavy people in the grocery store are the people with diet soda and processed food in the shopping cart?

Attention Alert: High Fructose Corn Syrup is not recognized by the human body as food and is therefore stored as fat.

The Sad Facts: Our conventional food supply contains an estimated 10,000 food additives, in addition to GMO ingredients and GMO fresh produce. Conventional factory farming makes wide use of pesticides, resulting in nutrient depleted farmlands and produce. Given all this, one has to marvel that the human body sustains itself as well as it does!

Given all this, one has to marvel that the human body sustains itself as well as it does!

Like food that contains hidden dairy ingredients, many foods also contain different types of sugars, each with its own name (Of course, by definition, any product with the word sugar, including date sugar, caster sugar, and coconut sugar, are indeed sugar products. By familiarizing yourself with this list, you'll further educate yourself with many other forms of sugars.

Agave

Agave Nectar

Anhydrous Dextrose

Cane Crystals

Cane Juice

Cane Juice Solids

Cane Syrup

Carbitol

Carob Syrup

Concentrated Fruit Juice

Confectioners' Sugar

Corn Sweetener

Corn Syrup

Corn Syrup Solids

Crystal Dextrose

Crystalline Fructose

Dehydrated Cane Juice

Dextran

Dextrose

Diglycerides

Disaccharides

Erythritol

Evaporated Cane Juice

Evaporated Cane Syrup

Florida Crystals

Fructooligosaccharides

Fructose

Fructose Crystals

Fructose Sweetener

Fruit juice Concentrate

Fruit juice Crystals

Galactose

Glazing Sugar

Glucitol

Glucoamine

Glucose

Glucose Syrup

Golden Sugar

Golden Syrup

Hexitol

(High-fructose Corn Syrup) (HFCS)

Honey

Icing

Inversol

Invert Syrup

Isomalt

King's Syrup

Lactose

Liquid Fructose

Malt Syrup

Maltose

Malted Barley

Maltodextrin

Maltose

Malts

Mannitol

Maple Syrup

Molasses

Muscovado

Nectar

Nectars

Pancake Syrup

Panocha

Pentose

Raisin Syrup

Sucrose

Refiners' Syrup

Sorghum

Ribose Rice Syrup

Rice Malt

Rice Syrup Solids

Sorbitol

Sorghum

Sorghum Syrup

Sucanat

Sucrose

Syrup

Treacle

Fructose

White sugar

Xylitol

Zylose

Getting To Know Your Healthy Sweeteners

Note: Some of the most healthful sweeteners are organic, raw, and unprocessed. These include raw honey, maple syrup, and black strap molasses.

Organic Raw Blue Agave is also a good sweetener choice. Like many of the other healthful sweeteners, the dark color is indicative of less processing. Agave has a very low glycemic load, which is certainly positive. However, it is also very high in fructose, which can cause insulin issues over time when consumed in high quantities and if not combined with high fiber and/or high fat foods. Try topping sweet potatoes, yam pie and coconut cream with a little organic Raw Blue Agave. Yum!

Stevia is great to grow in a garden because it grows like a weed! We make leaf sandwiches by placing one leaf of stevia between two peppermint leaves. This is not only delicious, but also serves as a breath freshener.

Avoid Artificial Sweeteners

Many experts believe that artificial sweeteners are *even worse* than sugar! Studies have connected artificial sweeteners with long-term undesirable health consequences. Additionally, they, too, are not recognized by the body as food. You can avoid consuming these artificial sweeteners by familiarizing yourself with their names and carefully reading labels.

ASPARTAME
APM
AminoSweet (but not in US)
Aspartyl-phenylalanine-1-methyl ester
Canderel (not in US)
Equal Classic
NatraTaste Blue
NutraSweet

ASPARTAME-ACESULFAME SALT
TwinSweet (Europe only)

CYCLAMATE
Not in US as per FDA
Calcium cyclamate
Cologran = cyclamate and

saccharin; not in US
Sucaryl

ERYTHRITOL
Sugar alcohol
Zerose
ZSweet

GLYCEROL
Glycerin
Glycerine

GLYCYRRHIZIN
Licorice

HYDROGENATED STARCH HYDROLYSATE (HSH)
Sugar alcohol

ISOMALT
Sugar alcohol
ClearCut Isomalt
Decomalt
DiabetiSweet (also contains
Acesulfame-K)
Hydrogenated Isomaltulose
Isomaltitol

LACTITOL
Sugar alcohol

MALTITOL
Sugar alcohol
Maltitol Syrup
Maltitol Powder
Hydrogenated High Maltose
Content Glucose Syrup
Hydrogenated Maltose
Lesys
MaltiSweet (hard to find
online to buy)
SweetPearl

MANNITOL
Sugar alcohol

NEOTAME

POLYDEXTROSE
Sugar alcohol
(Derived from glucose and
sorbitol)

SACCHARIN
Acid saccharin
Equal Saccharin
Necta Sweet
Sodium Saccharin
Sweet N Low
Sweet Twin

SORBITOL
Sugar alcohol
D-glucitol
D-glucitol syrup

SUCRALOSE
1',4,6'-
Trichlorogalactosucrose
Trichlorosucrose
Equal Sucralose
NatraTaste Gold
Splenda

TAGATOSE
Natrulose
XYLITOL
Sugar alcohol
Smart Sweet
Xylipure
Xylosweet

CHAPTER FIVE

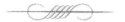

Getting Back To Basics: Sources, Markets & Making Selections

Cooking Equipment: Let's Get Back To Basics!

Cast iron frying pans are a cooking treasure and have been around for generations; they actually add trace amounts of iron into our food, which is a good thing, especially if you are prone to anemia. When you buy them new, cast iron frying pans have to be seasoned so foods don't stick. Many people use lard or bacon fat to season their pans. I have successfully used ghee in my cast iron pans, which I place in a 200-degree oven for several days. The pans absorb the fat so food easily slides off. With my next new cast iron frying pan, I'll try seasoning with unflavored coconut oil. Check my YouTube channel in the future to learn how well it works.

Stainless steel copper bottom pots, such as Revere Cookware, are standard issue and last for generations. CorningWare and other ceramic cookware are also good choices.

Do you use a microwave? Replace it with a Breville Convection Smart Oven. Microwave ovens use left-spinning energy to shake up the molecules that create heat. Left-spinning energy depletes life force. All living things have right spinning energy. The goal is to maintain life force, not deplete it!

All the items listed above are available at www.HealthyLivingWithDeirdre.com/Marketplace

Avoid Heavy Metals, Especially Aluminum

If you have aluminum or Teflon pots and pans, repurpose them as scrap metal. They have a high concentration of heavy metals that are toxic to your health. Aluminum is a cumulative poison and is known to be found in the autopsy reports of the deceased who have suffered from Alzheimer's.

The featured documentary, *The Age of Aluminum*, reveals the "dark side" of this toxic metal, exploring the scientific links between aluminum and diseases such as breast cancer and neurological disorders.

According to The Center for Disease Control, (CDC), *the average adult in the US consumes about seven-to-nine mg. of aluminum per day in food, and a lesser amount from air and water.*

You will be surprised at how much aluminum is in our food supply. Most factories while processing foods use equipment made from aluminum that leek into our food supply. Many processed foods actually list aluminum or forms thereof, such as aluminum chloride, as an ingredient. Examples of foods that might contain aluminum include baby formula, salt, baked goods, and anything packaged or stored in aluminum, so beware of water bottles and canned beverages. Personal care items such as cosmetics, deodorant, shampoo also often contain aluminum. Many drugs and antacids contain aluminum as well. The list is very long, adding bit by bit to the human consumption of aluminum.

Bottom line, avoid as best you can all contact with aluminum. First, eliminate aluminum foil and tins used for cooking and storing food. Instead, buy and store beverages in glass or stainless steel. Be mindful that often factories are using aluminum equipment to prepare foods.

And then there is baking powder. Baking powder is a mixture of sodium bicarbonate and cream of tartar, used instead of yeast in baking. When combined with wet ingredients, it acts as a leavening agent and adds fluffiness to baked goods. Also, be sure to use aluminum-free baking powder when baking. When buying baked goods, look for aluminum-free baking powder as an ingredient.

My favorite baking powder is: Rumford Aluminum Free Baking Powder.

Available:
www.HealthyLivingWithDeirdre.com/Marketplace
& Whole Foods

Loss Leaders Or Low Quality Food Products Are Often Discounted—Beware Of Coupons!

From time to time we all visit grocery stores. You know the kind, the big chain grocery store, sometimes with an emerging, although limited, organic section.

I was in line at the grocery store register, and there was a very friendly woman in front of me. She had a shopping cart full to the brim. She handed what looked like a four-inch stack of coupons to the cashier. This shopper saved a whopping $55 with that stack of coupons, and her bill was just over $60. Amazing! And then I began reviewing the items as they were packed into bags. There was not one item that I would actually consider "food," never mind that I would consider eating. Here is what occurred to me… If people decide to place the same effort they place in saving money, and redirect that effort to actually being responsible and knowledgeable about the food they and their families consume, our life experience—and state of health—would be far different.

Generally speaking, coupons are not issued for fresh, nutritious food. I have never known the local farmer or artisan cheese maker, or the Amish farmer, or the local winery or even Trader, to print and distribute coupons. These coupon products are generally of such poor quality that they require advertising and promotion to remain on the shelves.

Sources And Markets:

CSA Organic Farms, Amish farmers, local farmers, www.HealthyLivingWithDeirdre/com/Marketplace, local organic markets and co-ops, Whole Foods, and Trader Joe's are just a few of the many holistic markets. Let us remember that the Plant and Pray Garden—listed below—is also a viable option.

The Plant And Pray Garden:

Requires Just Planting And Watering—Test Drive Your Maintenance-Free Garden

In the spring and early summer, visit your local nursery garden centers or even mega stores such as Home Depot to buy organic or non-GMO heirloom seeds and seedlings. The selections will be the plants that grow in your area. If you are in a climate with four distinct seasons, you will find different selections in the early spring, then in the late spring /early summer. There are also many perennial vegetables, such as asparaguses and artichokes that do well in the cooler, four season climates. Plant them once, and they will return each year. Many herbs like oregano and mint will return each year. Also, if you'd like to try garlic, or a different bulb, plant them in the fall and they will be ready to harvest the following spring.

Other on-line catalog sources for available plants and seedlings include:

www.SeedsofChange.com   www.chileplants.com
www.teritorialseed.com   ww.kitchengardenseeds.com

How To Grow Your Garden:

Take small sections of your yard that perhaps have ground cover or grass along the edge of the planting areas and experiment. I plant, pray and water. Just let the plants do their thing! Herbs and certain vegetables, such as onions, scallions and chives, are essentially desirable weeds and will return each year after planting. Herbs and spices such as mint, oregano, basil, sage, parsley, cilantro, bay leaves, chives, scallions, stevia and chili peppers, all grow wild. Plant them all over the edge of your yard or in traditional unglazed clay pots. Mint especially spreads aggressively, so if you prefer to contain it to a particular area, pots are a good choice. Sometimes I bury a clay pot in the earth to contain the plant and yet have a natural manicured appearance without the effort. Yellow pear and grape tomatoes also do well in clay pots.

Based on their performance you will learn what area of the yard your plantings like the best. Toss in a few melons, tomatoes, sweet peppers, zucchini and cucumbers or whatever tickles your fancy.

Have you ever seen a tiny weed growing between bricks or a crack in concrete or something growing in a teaspoon of soil? It doesn't take much; the plant does most of the work. Plants will do everything to grow; the hardier the plant, the more nutrition and life force it contains!

Harvest in the late afternoon or evening and then water before dark. You will be surprised how much will grow with very little care. You can even forget about weeding and fertilizing. Just have fun!

How To Select Produce By The Number, By Reading Those Tiny Stickers!

Sticker numbers—also known as PLU codes—tell much about how a food is grown. Codes that begin with "4" mean the fruit or vegetable is grown "conventionally," with the use of pesticides. This also means that the soil is depleted of minerals and the food is nutritionally much less profitable. Codes that begin with "8" indicate the fruit or vegetable is genetically engineered. Be careful!

Genetically Modified Foods: Insights From A Brief History

The first commercially available genetically modified food was a tomato engineered to have a longer shelf life: the Flavr Savr. In 1994, the Flavr Savr was granted a license for human consumption.

The Flavr Savr failed to achieve commercial success and was withdrawn from the market in 1997. This is evidence of how voting with your dollar always makes a difference!

Another early tomato was developed that contained an antifreeze gene (*afa3*) from the winter flounder. The aim, here, was to increase the tomato's tolerance to frost. This genetic modification caused quite a stir in the early years of the debate over genetically modified foods, especially in relation to the perceived ethical dilemma of combining genes from different species.

BBC News in 1999 stated it would be six years before certain GMO glowing potatoes would be available for sale. When announced, the researchers had done more than three years of laboratory experiments and soon anticipated started field trials. However, to date, environmental activists have worked to prevent field tests.

The Rationale for Genetically Modified Jellyfish Potatoes: Science has shown that when potato crops do not get sufficient water, the yield can be reduced by up to two thirds. At present, farmers have no reliable method to test whether their crops have adequate water, except to wait for signs of wilting. Scientists have genetically modified potatoes so that they glow when they need watering. Prof Trewavas and his team created the 'intelligent' potato by adding a gene from the jellyfish, Aequorea Victoria. Triggered by a protein that forms as the plant becomes dehydrated, this jellyfish gene causes the leaves to glow.

For more information about the tomato fish story and other related news effecting our food supply visit: www.motherearthnews.com or OrganicConsumersAssociation.com

Theoretically, there could be flounder DNA in your tomato or jellyfish DNA in your potatoes! With GMO foods, you have no way of knowing what you are actually consuming! Incidentally, genetically engineered food is banned in Europe. Some research shows that genetically engineered foods cause unusual autoimmune responses and systemic inflammation. Of course, it's your choice whether to buy these foods, but for me, it's simply not worth the risk. Rather, look for codes that begin with 9. These are organically grown, high nutritional content foods. By the way, the last three digits merely indicate the type of fruit or vegetable.

Note: When selecting produce, you might want to keep this rhyme in mind:

Number 4, think some more;

Number 8, definitely NOT great;

Number 9 is divine.

CHAPTER SIX

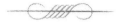

Water Quality Always Matters! Especially In High Water Content Foods, Like Fruit

USDA Organic - Lack Of Standards For Water Quality Used For Irrigation.

"The USDA organic regulations do not directly address the use of irrigation water on organic farms." A direct quote from the spokesman for the USDA's National Organics Program.

Unfortunately, current labeling often does not tell us what farm the produce came from. Fracking wastewater continues to be an issue in some areas, contaminating and /or being used as irrigation water on USDA organic farms. We must be mindful of the drought conditions in many agricultural regions. The good news is you can taste the difference. My favorite high water content fresh produce comes from farms that utilize underground aquifers or rainwater, rather than irrigation. To stay up to date on these and many other issues affecting our food supply and our home planet Earth visit www.organicconsumers.org.

All Life Depends On Water, And Alkaline Water = High Quality Life And Good Health

I cannot stress enough the importance of drinking high quality water and using high quality water in our farms and homes. You have to be drinking alkaline water. Water should be stored in glass or stainless steel containers. The PH should be as high above seven as possible, say PH 8 or 9. This can be accomplished three ways:

(1) Create high quality water with a counter top reverse osmosis water filter system. You drink the alkaline water and you can use the acidic water waste for cleaning.

(2) Purchase alkaline water at shops like Phountain, a lifestyle detox establishment that sells alkaline water and other services and is now offering national franchising opportunities, or

(3) Make your own. The higher the PH, the higher your blood's oxygen content will be. The higher the oxygen content the more energy and healing power your body enjoys. Did you know that actuaries have already determined that people who live at sea level live longer? This is because at sea level the oxygen content is higher in the air we breathe than at higher altitudes. The Harbor Rose, our B&B located in Cold Spring Harbor, NY, serves solarized alkaline water in blue bottles made from purified water. Our guests notice the difference. You will too!

Taking into account water quality and the environment, I believe the best solution is installing a water filter system in your home and place of business. There are several reverse osmosis filter systems on the market for both on the counter and under the counter. Perhaps consider installing a water filter system in your entire house like we have at The Harbor Rose. Alternatively, the simplest least expensive option is to make your own alkaline water with the sun-solarized system; it will be an upgrade to tap water even if you make it with unfiltered tap water. People all over the world that don't have running water have been using the sun to purify water for generations. It works.

How To Make Your Own Solarized Alkaline Water

Locate several large glass bottles. My favorites are cobalt blue / dark blue glass bottles such as a SKYY vodka bottles. Fill them with tap water and place them in the sun with no top for 3 - 4 hours: the longer, the better. The lower the quality of water you are starting with the more sun time required. Experiment and you will find what works best for you. Using the sun to purify your water increases the alkalinity. If it's too cold outside or you don't have access to sunlight on a particular day; use a traditional incandescent 60-watt light bulb and place the bottles underneath the lamp. Let them stay for a minimum of five hours. You'll be amazed how good this water tastes.

> Chapped lips are a sign of dehydration. The cure? Drink more high quality water!

Water And Energy

Water absorbs energy and can be re-imprinted any time. Perhaps this is the reason why religious leaders and some adherents bless water rather than rocks or dirt. For more information about water you might explore Dr. Masaru Emoto's work and read his book, *The Secret Messages in Water.* In short, he has found that water retains memory imprints from thoughts, music, and labels. I have expanded on Dr. Emoto's work, as he has established scientific evidence that water retains memory and can be re-imprinted by environmental factors.

I am conceptually taking his work a step further based on my background and understanding of the healing arts of ancient cultures and homeopathic medicine. Homeopathic Medicine was founded in the late 1700s in Germany and is widely used in Europe. (Perhaps this is one reason that their health care costs are so much lower than the US, but that's for another time!) One of the basic principals in Homeopathic Medicine is "energy frequencies." The "energy frequencies" of healthy tissue are different from the "energy frequencies" of unhealthy tissue. With the right energy frequencies, balance can be restored and the body healed. An example of this is a trained human voice that, while generating the correct frequency, can shatter a glass. The correct homeopathic energy frequency can shatter or transform a pathogen in the same way, healing the body. In basic terms, here is the concept. If you have chlorinated water and the chlorine is filtered out, the "memory" of the chlorine remains in the water; more specifically, you have not filtered out the "energy frequency" of the chlorine that was in the water. We are imprinting the "energy frequencies" in the water by using blue bottles and sunlight.

Drugs In Our Water Supply?

Pharmaceuticals Drugs In Our Water Supply

In addition to the pollutants, much of the US population is consuming pharmaceuticals. These pharmaceuticals, or perhaps even their "energy frequencies," are showing up in our water supply, another reason for drinking and cooking with solarized water made from purified water.

This issue was brought to light in 2008 when these findings and studies were (first) published. Traces of cancer and psychiatric drugs were found in Britain's tap water, according to a 100-page report commissioned by the Drinking Water Inspectorate (DWI).

Jeff Donn, Maratha Mendoza and Justin Pritchard of the Associated Press reported the following study-based findings: "A vast array of pharmaceuticals including antibiotics, anti-convulsants, mood stabilizers and sex hormones have been found in the drinking water supplies of at least 41 million Americans, an Associated Press investigation shows."

Dr. Janssen, a researcher, speaks to WebMD: "Contamination is not confined to the United States. More than 100 different pharmaceuticals have been detected in lakes, rivers, reservoirs and streams throughout the world. Studies have detected pharmaceuticals in waters throughout Asia, Australia, Canada and

Europe, even in Swiss lakes and the North Sea, and is affecting wildlife." She adds that, "Concern among scientists increased when fish in the Potomac River and elsewhere were found to have both male and female characteristics when exposed to estrogen-like substances. For instance, some fish had both testes and an ovary."

Interestingly, to date there is no governmental oversight on "levels" of drugs in our water supply. Given the aforementioned study results, and multiple others, I strongly recommend that you take matters into your own hands. (See Aforementioned Water Systems). To my knowledge, bottled water companies do not test for pharmaceuticals. Some researchers also claim that the plastic in water bottles leaches into the water. Finally, as mentioned previously, it's best to drink alkaline water to help balance the body's alkalinity. Many spring water sources are alkaline neutral. By drinking solarized and purified water, you'll empower yourself, improve your health, and also help the environment!

CHAPTER SEVEN

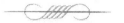

The ROYGBIV Rainbow Guide To High Profit Alkaline Foods

Eat Every Color Every Day—it's easier than you think!

Food Colors provide insight into the nutrients contained in the food.

Have you ever asked a young child what he or she has had for lunch and received a blank stare? I certainly have! But when asked, what colors did you eat for lunch, boy do the same children remember, and with a great deal of enthusiasm! There is a child inside each and every one of us who can remember what colors we consume each day. Give it a try today. When you eat each color represented in the rainbow, you are consuming high profit, high nutrition foods.

The freshest and highest quality produce is sourced from your CSA Organic Farm Membership and your Plant and Pray Garden, followed by local organic farmers' markets, Whole Foods or Trader Joe's.

A Bit About Potatoes And Yams

There are countless varieties of potatoes, a type of root vegetable that stores very well. You can tell which of these are most profitable by their color! Select purple, garnet, Japanese or Hanna yams, blue potatoes, and ruby sensation potatoes. Yukon gold, russet, fingerling, red and Idaho potatoes are the least nutritious. That said, a small red potato is very useful in making vegan soups. They are also commonly used for potato salad because of their high moisture content. My favorite in the potato family are yams, for their high nutrition and low glycemic load. Japanese yams and purple yams are also great for making French fries and mashed potatoes!

Shopping Tip: When shopping for groceries, buy what you expect to consume in three days. Keep it simple. Look at the cart, is the rainbow evenly represented?

Color Overview: Let's Start With Red
Red foods support joint tissue health, reduces bad cholesterol, lower blood pressure, protect the body from free radicals, and reduce the risk of many cancers. They are packed with vitamin A and C, Lycopene, and many other valuable nutrients. Consider incorporating into your diet the following, nutritious red foods:

Red Fruit Cherries:

Red fruit cherries are very soothing and calming and high in fiber.

Available frozen at Trader Joe's & Whole Foods.

Raspberries & Strawberries:

Raspberries and strawberries have seeds on the outside of the skin. This is the first clue of their powerful antioxidant and detoxifying properties. Seeds on the outside of the fruit push toxins out of your body through your skin. Many people are allergic to strawberries. The allergy may not be a fruit allergy, but rather an allergy to the pesticides used by conventional strawberry growers. It's always preferable to buy fresh, organic berries. If fresh organic berries are not in your budget, strawberry growers. It's always preferable to buy fresh organic berries.

Trader Joe's has nice frozen options. If you are buying fresh and can't find organic berries, your best choices are berries grown in Europe or the USA.

Available frozen at Trader Joe's and Whole Foods.

Red Vegetables

Carrots:

These root vegetables come in a variety of colors. Why not try a red carrot?

Raw foods provide enzymes for digestive health and improve elimination. Try raw carrots dipped into hummus for a fun appetizer.

Trader Joe's has been carrying bags of fresh rainbow carrots. Slice them into similar sizes and steam. Serve with a bit of white truffle oil and pink Himalayan sea salt. Sprinkle some fresh chopped chives or marjoram and serve—just divine!

Shopping tip: Trader Joe's has been stocking organic rainbow carrots.

White Truffle oil is available at www.TheCrushedOlive.com.

Sweet Peppers: Enjoy these tasty treats sliced raw or slightly sautéed. Peppers are packed with vitamins and minerals that support weight management. Keep a bag of frozen assorted color peppers on hand for a quick soup or chili.

Available at Trader Joe's.

Tomatoes: Tomatoes are actually a fruit, not a vegetable. They are both low in calories and are an anti-cancer, anti-aging food, filled with healthful nutrients. My favorites are grape tomatoes, and all the heirloom varieties available in summer. In the winter, enjoy Kumato tomatoes; these brown tomatoes are full of flavor. Tomatoes are actually a fruit, not a vegetable. They are both low in calories and are an anti-cancer, anti-aging food, filled with healthful nutrients. My favorites are grape tomatoes, and all the heirloom varieties available in summer. In the winter, enjoy Kumato tomatoes; these brown tomatoes are full of flavor. Remember to keep them on the counter rather than the fridge. Room temperature maintains the rich flavors!

Available at Trader Joe's & Whole Foods

Let's Eat Orange

Overview

Beta carotene is what gives orange foods their color. These foods contain retinal, retinol and retinoic acid, which are full of vitamins A and C, especially important for night vision. These antioxidants can neutralize the damaging free radicals in the body and are crucial for a healthy immune system. Orange foods also protect against cardiovascular disease and help rebuild your skin collagen.

Orange food is a great choice to do a quick test on your digestive track. For an entire day, eat only orange food. On the day's menu include garnet yams, carrots, red lentils, orange tomatoes, orange peppers and orange citrus. To ascertain if your digestive track is in good order, your urine should be the same color as the foods that you consumed: purely orange. If that's not the case, this is a good indication that you need to clean your digestive track. The gut-flushed diet is a good way to accomplish cleaning and rebalancing your intestinal flora in order to help restore your immune system. A great book with an effective protocol is *The Gut Flush Plan* by Ann Louise.

Available: www.HealthyLivingWithDeirdre.com/Marketplace

Orange Fruit

Cantaloupe	This delicious melon contains a wide variety of antioxidant and anti-inflammatory phytonutrients and vitamins. I tried them in my Plant and Pray Garden, with a variety that matures in 60 days into small personal size melons—they are so cute and delicious!
Oranges:	This popular fruit is rich in vitamin C and other nutrients. My favorites are the easy peel navel oranges. Clementines or Halos are also a nice easy peel without getting sticky fingers and are small enough for a child's lunch box. I prefer citrus from

Florida for several reasons. Citrus is a high water content food. We already know that organic standards have no jurisdiction when it comes to the quality of water used in organic farming. We also know that fracking is an issue when it comes to water quality. As I'm writing this, fracking is not permitted in the state of Florida, although many are working to overturn this decision. Florida also has hard water, high mineral content, and we are always seeking the highest nutrition available.

Orange Vegetables

Butternut Squash: Butternut squash is a very healthy sweet squash that is great for soups and a winter favorite. It is high in fiber and phytonutrients as well as vital poly-phenolic anti-oxidants and vitamins. Peel and remove seeds, cut into cubes and steam. It's also nice mashed as a side dish. I like it seasoned with turmeric and cinnamon.

Carrots: This root vegetable is high in beta-carotene, an important antioxidant, and a good source of fiber. It also aids in controlling blood pressure, hunger, and, as previously mentioned, is good for eye health. Great raw when you just feel like chewing!

Garnet Yams: These yams are sweet tasting, low in sugars, high in fiber and high quality carbs, high in vitamins C and A and in calcium and iron. I enjoy this variety fried in coconut oil and served with mustard.

Orange Tomatoes: Ever try the small, round, orange cherry tomatoes? Great for the Plant and Pray Garden and oh so sweet!

Sweet Peppers: Sweet bell peppers add color to every dish. Remember to enjoy them raw as well as cooked.

It's Time for Yellow
Overview:

Yellow fruits and vegetables are abundant in vitamin C, carotenoids and bioflavonoids, which function as antioxidants. These nutrients support heart heath, vision, digestion and one's immune system. Other benefits include maintenance of healthy skin and stronger bones and teeth.

Yellow Fruit:
Lemons: This citrus fruit is delicious, especially when you squeeze one whole lemon into your alkaline water daily. Add a bit of maple syrup if you desire it a bit sweeter. Lemons are packed with vitamins C, A and B complex. Lemons also contain a variety ofphytochemicals. Hesperetin, naringin, and naringenin are flavonoid glycosides commonly found in citrus fruits. Naringenin is found to have a bio-active effect on human health as an antioxidant, free radical scavenger, anti-inflammatory, and immune system modulator. Lemons contain vitamin A, also required for maintaining healthy

mucus membranes, skin and essential for vision. Lemons are rich in flavonoids that help to protect the body from lung and oral cavity cancers and many other chronic diseases, including arthritis, obesity and coronary heart disease. Let's not forget about beneficial minerals such as iron, copper, potassium, and calcium. Potassium is an important component of cell and body fluids that help control heart rate and blood pressure. When I select lemons, I favor the soft squishy ones, as they are juicer! I also find that at times the organic ones are less expensive than the non-organic. Sometimes non-organic lemons are sold by the piece and the organic, by weight. Try tossing a few organic lemons onto the scale at the market, and compare prices. You might be surprised.

Mango: This amazingly delicious and healthy fruit comes in many varieties. The mango contains abundant antioxidant compounds found to protect against colon, breast, leukemia and prostate cancers. These compounds include quercetin, isoquercitrin, astragalin, fisetin, gallic acid and methylgallat, as well as abundant enzymes. Mangos offer twenty different vitamins and minerals. My favorite variety is Organic Madame Francique mangoes from Haiti. They are quite large and have a growing season from April – August.

Available: Whole Foods

Pineapple: This bountiful fruit supports heart heath. It is high in fiber, potassium and vitamin C and contains bromelain, a wonderful enzyme commonly used to treat sprains, tendinitis, and minor muscle issues because it reduces inflammation.

Yellow Watermelon: This version is just as delicious as the red version and comes in small, personalized sizes.

Yellow Vegetables Corn and Baby Corn: Can you differentiate between these two? Baby corn is regular corn that has not matured. When in season, it's available fresh at Whole Foods. The baby corn is much lower in sugars, lower in carbs, and higher in fiber than mature corn. It's a good source of iron and other essential nutrients. You often find them canned in Asian markets, and Native Forest has a canned organic version. Trader Joe's offers a frozen organic super sweet corn, which is delicious. Prepare it like the peas, defrosted but not cooked! Toss a bit into salads or soups to balance the glycemic load.

Available: www.HealthyLivingWithDeirdre/com/Mark etplace, Whole foods & Trader Joe's

Golden Beets: Like other root vegetables, Golden Beets are very grounding and don't have the strong, earthy flavor of red beets. Golden or yellow beets are heart healthy, excellent kidney and body cleansers, and high in powerful antioxidants. They also lower blood pressure and cholesterol, and treat anemia and fatigue. They are associated with a reduced risk of heart disease and help in the prevention of various cancers. They are also good for eyes and skin.

Yellow Tomatoes: These tomatoes have many of the same benefits as all the other tomatoes, and are also less acidic tasting then the red varieties. My favorites are the small, pear-shaped tomatoes. They are very sweet and the appealing shape looks lovely on a plate. They grow well in containers in your Plant and Pray Garden; this plant delivers an abundance of fruit. Yellow pear tomatoes are a great item for toddlers as they are small and sweet.

Sweet Peppers: These peppers are high in vitamins C, B-6, Folate, A, Thiamin, Niacin and B-5. They're also high in minerals, including iron, magnesium, phosphorus, potassium and copper. They are fresh and crunchy and great raw. You're sure to notice the difference in flavor when selecting organic vs conventional.

Don't Forget Your Greens!

Overview:

Chlorophyll is a pigment that provides the green color, but it offers so much more. Chlorophyll naturally takes carbon dioxide and converts it into oxygen. In short, green vegetables are naturally detoxifying, and very important for a healthy respiratory system. They also naturally increase your energy level and improve your digestive track. Fruits and vegetables that grow on vines contribute creative energies to our systems, so be sure to enjoy some!

Avocado: Commonly believed to be a vegetable, an avocado is actually a fruit. It contains high amounts of healthy fats that support brain function. The fiber supports waste elimination and the fruit itself is a good source of protein. Consume three or four a week! You can use avocado as a mayo replacement or make some guacamole and serve with blue corn chips. You will eat fewer chips for sure! Simply mash the avocado, add some fresh squeezed lemon or lime juice, finely chopped tomato, onion, and cilantro and jalapeno peppers to taste. (If you find these peppers too spicy remove the seeds and enjoy only the flesh.) My favorite avocados are organic haas. They are firmer in texture than other varieties and, in my experience, the organic ones often times have smaller pits and more fruit.

Available at Trader Joe's & Whole Foods

Green Grapes: Although green grapes are tasty, taking into account calories and nutritional content, you get more "bang for your buck" and profit by choosing black, blue Thompson, concord grapes or even red grapes over green grapes. If you choose to purchase green grapes, it's best to choose   those with the darkest, rich green color available. These citrus fruits are naturally alkalizing and delicious in water when fresh squeezed. We always have a dozen or so limes on hand for special drinks. Each serving contains one lime squeezed into alkaline water with crushed ice and just a dash of maple syrup, and, in the summertime a sprig of mint from the Plant and Pray Garden. It's yummy and festive!

Vegetables
Lettuce and
Salad Greens: The most common and the least nutritious lettuce is light green iceberg lettuce, although it is better than no lettuce at all! A good rule of thumb when selecting lettuce is the darker the green, the greater the nutritional benefits. Also, darker green lettuce that contains red and purple is even more chock full of nutrients.

Some of my favorite types of lettuce include red leaf Boston lettuce, sometimes called butter lettuce. When choosing lettuce, explore new-looking leaves; all baby greens are tender and sweet. The best source of fresh greens is your local CSA organic farm or your Plant and Pray Garden, as this will be the freshest source.

The Time Saver: Herb Blend Baby Field Greens is a pre-washed, tasty lettuce blend. My favorite is Earthbound Farm Organic Herb Blend.

Available at Whole Foods

The Short Cut: E3 Live: Don't like salad or green leafy vegetables? No problem. Take two table-spoons of E3 Live a day. It comes in a plastic bottle and can be found in the frozen department of Whole Foods, or perhaps your local organic market. Defrost the liquid and place into single serving ice cube trays. Defrost a cube each day and drink it. This is especially effective if you feel the beginning of a cold; E3 Live will help nip it in the bud.

Available: www.HealthyLivingWithDeirdre.com/Marketplace

The Quickie:
Blue Green Algae: Found in capsules, these supplements are training wheels for those who are experimenting with different ways to obtain better nutrition. Nature's Way has chlorella that is non-GMO and made with 100% Vegetarian Capsules. Available: www.HealthyLivingWithDeirdre/com/Marketplace, Whole Foods.

Other Green Vegetables

Green Beans: Also known as string beans and pole beans, green beans come in many varieties and are easy items for the Plant and Pray garden because they don't require full sun. These beans are high in vitamins A and K, which is good for bone and eye health and contain cholesterol-lowering fiber. Eat them raw or gently steamed. My personal favorites are the French style uncut, a small thin bean.

A nonorganic version is available at Trader Joe's.

Broccoli/
Brussels Sprouts: These two green vegetables reduce the risk of developing cancer by increasing glucosinolate in the body. Both are high in fiber and low in calories.

Brussels sprouts are rich in many valuable nutrients including vitamins C and K. They are also a good source of numerous nutrients, including folate, manganese, vitamin B6, dietary fiber, choline, copper, vitamin B1, potassium, phosphorus, and omega-3 fatty acids. I like them steamed until they are bright green and served with goat butter and pink Himalayan sea salt.

Broccoli also contains vitamins A (in the form carotenoids) B1, B5, B6, C, and K, chromium, folate and fiber, manganese, phosphorus, choline, potassium, and copper.

I always peel my broccoli stalks; the flower, and the stem cook at the same rate. I just peel the thick skin with a paring knife. Check my YouTube for a demonstration.

Celery: When buying celery, always choose organic. The important nutrients in celery are in its natural high mineral content. Conventional celery has little to no minerals as the soil has been depleted of nutrients (a byproduct of factory farming), so unless you buy organic you will not enjoy the natural salty flavor of real celery. If you find yourself adding salt to your food, this is evidence of your body requiring and asking for minerals. Organic celery is naturally salty due to its high mineral content, so use more celery when cooking or toss it into your salad. It's also a great source of vitamins A, K, and C, folate, potassium, dietary fiber, as well as flavonoids, which decrease inflammation and blood clots and are known to reduce blood pressure. Although not dark green, celery is an important, high profit food.

Cucumbers: This wonderful vegetable is cooling to the body, so it's a great choice on a hot day! It is also a good source of vitamin A, pantothenic acid, magnesium, phosphorus and manganese, and a great source of vitamin C, vitamin K and potassium. My favorites are Persian and English varieties. Cucumbers are great for the Plant and Pray Garden. While only the skin is dark green, cucumbers are so full of nutrition and so easy to enjoy, I had to include them in this book.

Available at Trader Joe's and Whole Foods.

Peas: These little gems are a great source of protein, one of the highest protein content vegetables. They are hard to find organic and fresh unless you try growing them in your Plant and Pray Garden. However, Trader Joe's has frozen petite peas. Give them a try. Simply pour some into a strainer and pour boiling water over them so they defrost, but don't cook. Add a little Himalayan pink salt to these deliciously sweet treats and enjoy! I also find that toddlers enjoy them frozen.

Trader Joe's Brand Petite Peas – frozen
Available: Trader Joe's

Zucchini: Although zucchini is not one of the high profit foods, I felt it was important to include because this "in demand" vegetable is, unfortunately, one of the vegetables that is often GMO. Be sure to buy organic when selecting zucchini. My favorite variety has the dark green skin. Zucchini is another great item for the Plant and Pray Garden.

Serving suggesting: Make zucchini pasta by peeling the entire zucchini with a potato peeler into strips that resemble linguini pasta. In a pot, place some olive oil, finely chopped garlic, and tomato sauce. Then add the zucchini on top. Stir on a very low heat until the zucchini wilts down (just a few minutes) and serve with some parsley garnish. It's delicious!

Blue/ Indigo / Violet – Three Colors Of The Rainbow!

Overview:
Here's the good news! An analysis of the latest data from the National Health and Nutrition Examination Study (NHANES), a survey of eating and health habits, found that adults who eat purple

and blue fruits and vegetables have reduced risk for both high blood pressure and obesity. They also benefit from higher levels of HDL cholesterol (the "good" kind!)

Scientists believe that anthocyanins, compounds that give purple foods their color, are responsible for these boons. These anthocyanins are known for fighting fatigue, inflammation, short-term memory loss and stomach disorders, reducing risk of heart disease, keeping the eyes and urinary tract healthy and lowering the risk of gum disease and stomach ulcers. Blue and purple foods are rich in flavonoids. These compounds mop up free radicals and reduce inflammation. Purple foods also contain ellagic acid, a phytochemical that may be linked to cancer prevention and reducing cholesterol levels.

I suspect all Americans will benefit from increasing their purple and blue food intake. You will also find that most foods in this category are seasonally available. Is it really so bad to be connected to the seasons? As a society, we are always trying to control nature; how about benefitting from all it has to offer as a change of pace?

Purple Foods are Regenerative.

The regenerative power of purple foods is very evident when growing a garden. I was growing Japanese eggplant, and one morning when I went out to water, I noticed a large bite had been taken out of one of the eggplants. It had only grown about two thirds of the size, indicating its readiness to be picked. Interestingly, over time, the plant healed right over and continued growing and maturing. I don't know any other fruit or vegetable that grows this way. Purple food regenerates itself and it assists in your body regenerating cells when you eat it. So be sure to include lots of high profit purple foods in your diet!

Indigo / Blue / Purple Fruit

Acai: This true superfood is packed with nutrition and is available in frozen form. It's indigenous to the Brazilian Rainforest and is high in fats. Acai has a chocolate-like overtone in its flavor. Be sure to select brands without additional ingredients. Commonly used in smoothies, we enjoy it as an ice pop. My favorite brand is Sambazon Unsweetened Pure Açai Berry smoothie packs.

Available: www.HealthyLivingWithDeirdre.com/Mark etplace & Whole Foods

Bilberry Jam: This is a must try. I have not been able to find this delectable berry fresh in the US, but this jam is delicious. Bilberry extract has been given to fighter pilots to improve night vision. It is powerful. On occasion, I unintentionally ingest canola oil. Whenever I do so, my vision takes a dive. It's this jam alone, with lots of high quality water, which restores my vision. My favorite brand for jam is Bionaturae Organic Fruit Spread Bilberry. My favorite extract is Nature's Plus - Bilberry, 50 mg, 1 fl. Oz. liquid.

Available: www.HealthyLivingWithDeirdre.com/Mark etplace & Whole Foods

Black Grapes: These delicious grapes are often seedless, crunchy and store well. Slice them in half and add them to salads. These grapes help the body to produce collagen, and contain vitamins, calcium and iron. The skins of black seedless grapes contain compounds that benefit your health. Research published in January 2011 issue of the "Annals of the New York Academy of Sciences" notes that resveratrol in grapes may act as a therapeutic agent for severe acute pancreatitis, preventing its progression. Polyphenols in some seedless grapes may help decrease your risk of developing cancer, according to research in the 2008 "Journal of Environmental Pathology, Toxicology and Oncology."

Black Mission Figs:

These figs are deliciously sweet, super high in fiber, and a good source of several essential minerals, including magnesium, manganese, calcium (which promotes bone density), copper, and potassium (which helps lower blood pressure), as well as vitamins, principally K and B6. They are available fresh when in season at a reasonable price at Trader Joe's and Costco. When fresh, eat them when they are soft and squishy. Dried mission figs are available year round at Trader Joe's. If you choose the dried type, try steaming them a bit to plump them up. Figs are a nutrient-dense choice for snacks and/or an ingredient in baking recipes, and a great natural solution for constipation.

Available: Trader Joe's & Whole Foods

Note: Dried figs are often too dry for my taste and give a sense of chewing leather. However, wild and raw organic sun-dried figs, they are quite lovely.

Available: www.HealthyLivingWithDeirdre.com/Mark etplace & Whole Foods

Blackberries & Blueberries: Packed with nutrients, super high in fiber and low in natural sugars, these fruits are also delicious. Fresh is best, although frozen wild organic is available at Trader Joe's for a reasonable price. Both are packed with nutrients and powerful antioxidant properties. In 2011, blueberries made the Environmental Working Group's "Dirty Dozen" for their high pesticide content, so buy them organic as often as possible.

For frozen options, I recommend organic wild blueberries.

Available: at Trader Joe's.

Concord Grapes: These grapes come with seeds that are small and easy to digest. The September 2009 issue of "The Journal of Nutrition" reports that the phytochemicals and antioxidants in grape seeds have the ability to fight cancer and improve your overall health.
Unfortunately, since seedless grapes were introduced into the US market in the 1970s, seedless grapes represent 80% market share

in the US. While we do have grape seed extract in the marketplace, in keeping with my whole foods philosophy, I recommend purchasing the seeded grapes themselves. Indigenous to the northern regions of the US, concord grapes contain oligomeric proanthrocyanadin complexes—which the University of Maryland Medical Center says are powerful antioxidants—in addition to other nutrients such as vitamin-E, flavonoids and linoleic acids. Flavonoids are believed to lower the risk of heart disease by decreasing your body's concentration of LDL, or "bad" cholesterol. Additionally, according to the USDA Agricultural Research Service, polyphenols found in concord grapes and other foods can strengthen your immune response, heal damage that you may have sustained at the cellular level and could even protect you from developing some forms of cancer! When in season, concord grapes are readily available and delicious!

Black Plums: With their tart, black skin and sweet, deep-red flesh, these plums are not only juicy and delicious when in season, they're also nutritionally packed! Plums protect the intestinal track, help to manage high blood pressure, and contain nutrients that are associated with a reduced risk of death from all causes, including heart disease, stroke and cancer! Plums also help with the absorption of iron.

Black Olives: These olives provide heart healthy fat, anti-inflammatory elements, trace minerals, vitamin E, iron, potassium and fiber. They've also been found to lower cholesterol! Jared in olive oil is best, as canned olives are packed in water and salt. Soak canned olives in purified water to remove the sodium. One of my favorite varieties is Trader Joe's Pitted Kalamata Olives with extra virgin olive oil, in a jar.

Indigo / Blue / Purple Vegetables:

Purple Cabbage: Commonly known as red cabbage, purple cabbage is very low in calories, and has fat burning properties. It is an excellent source of vitamins K, C, and B6. It is also a very good source of manganese, dietary fiber, potassium, vitamin B1, folate and copper. As an added bonus, it stores well and is great for making coleslaw.

Purple Cauliflower: Available when in season and usually locally grown, purple cauliflower is high in fiber. The purple comes from anthocyanins, which are antioxidant flavonoids, naturally occurring plant pigments. These flavonoids hold potential health benefits, including the ability to help stabilize capillary walls. This is important because weak capillary walls allow toxic substances to permeate cells. A yummy way to serve it is to sauté it in gold label coconut oil with garlic and chili peppers.

CHAPTER EIGHT

High Quality Oils Are Important For Brain Function

Exchanging Low Quality Oils For Their Healthy Counterparts—Olive Oil, Coconut Oil, And Other Fats

High quality oils are critically important for brain function. High cholesterol is evidence of a low quality or low fat diet. Cholesterol is your body's survival strategy after suffering from years of consuming low quality fats and oils often found in low fat foods. Cholesterol is your body's spackle team, repairing cracks created by a loss of elasticity. As your arteries become brittle the spackle team comes in to patch things up, and your arteries become clogged. Adding high quality oils to your diet will help solve this problem.

Low quality oils include canola oil from a modified version of the rape seed plant. This is the plant 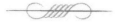 **90% of the US canola crop is GMO.** used to clean up contaminated toxic soil. Originally used as an industrial lubricant, even animals and insects avoid eating this plant. The oil was first added to animal feed. In the late 1980s, a man named John Thomas reported that canola oil, when fed to livestock in Europe, caused the animals to become aggressive towards people and each other. Worse, the animals began going blind. When the rapeseed derivative was removed from the diet of these sheep, pigs, and cows, the problems mysteriously disappeared. In 1991, after the findings were revealed in Thomas' book, *Young Again,* Europe banned the product. Then it appeared in the human food supply as cholesterol-free oil. It was given a new name—canola oil—and marketed as a "healthy oil." Because of its low price, it's in many products. I have had clients who use glasses actually get weaker prescriptions from the eye doctor after removing canola oil from their diet. Do your best to read labels and avoid this product.

Besides, there are healthful, high quality oils and fats from which to choose.

Butter: Most butter is made from cow milk. Look for rBST (from cows raised without growth hormones) organic butter. Amish butter is a good source for high quality cow milk-based butter. European style butter has less salt.

I highly recommend goat butter for so many reasons. You will notice a significant difference in taste; goat butter is not anywhere near a gamey taste as cow butter. Additionally, the small proteins in goat butter are much easier to digest. My favorite is European style Meyenberg goat butter, which is very tasty and freezes quite well. If you are interested in upgrading to this type of butter, be mindful that it is a seasonal product, available in the late spring, and can be bought in bulk.

Available: www.meyenberg.com

Tip: If the butter is out of stock or the shipping is too expensive, ask for the local distributor contact info. I have found that the local distributer has lower shipping costs.

Coconut Oil: There are countless benefits to coconut oil, upon which many books expound. Coconut oil is the best choice for high temperature cooking and frying, creating crispy food. If you think about it, this makes sense, since coconut palms are indigenous to high temperature climates around the equator, where temperatures often exceed 100°F. Coconut oil is also great for treating dry skin and very effective for chapped lips.

It is also important to note that coconut oil burns like a carbohydrate, fueling your body with energy. Unlike some other oils, this oil is not stored in fat tissue. When making a selection, seek organic and cold pressed, preferably hand pressed.

My favorite brand is Tropical Traditions. This company offers an expeller pressed flavored and unflavored high quality coconut oil, both of which are USDA organic. The flavored one is delicious; I often use it to sauté broccoli and cauliflower, Chinese style, which I season with a little chili pepper, garlic and herbs. The unflavored version is great for frying.

Cooking Tip: When frying vegetables, add a splash of water to reduce the cooking time.

Note: My preference is to purchase the gallon size, each of which comes in a bucket with a handle. The bucket can be used in so many ways—as a compost bucket for the kitchen counter, a holder of gardening tools, and for various projects.

The unflavored version is Expeller-Pressed Coconut Oil. The flavored version I recommend purchasing is Gold Label® Virgin Coconut Oil.

Available: www.HealthyLivingWithDeirdre.com/Marketplace & www.TropicalTraditions.com

Tip: If you have a crack in the crease of your upper and lower lip, you have a vitamin B2 deficiency. Lick a vitamin B2 tablet, and rub on the crack before swallowing. This will help the crack resolve.

Ghee: This is a great fat, commonly used in Indian cuisine. This clarified butter has no milk solids, only milk fat. "While most clarified butters are prepared by removing milk solids in early steps, ghee differentiates itself by continuing to simmer with the milk solids to give a final product with a distinguished taste," says registered dietitian Raman Khatar of "Food For Thought" in Vancouver. "And because of way it's prepared, the lactose and milk protein content is nil to minimal, making it better tolerated by those with dairy sensitivities."

It's a great replacement for butter, especially when cooking, as it does not burn. My preferred brand is Purity Farms Organic Chee.

Available: www.HealthyLivingWithDeirdre.com/Mark etplace & Whole Foods.

Olive Oil: It's best to use olive oil on already cooked or raw foods, such as fresh salads. Olive oil should never be cooked at high temperatures, which causes the long chain fatty acids to break down and creates harmful free radicals. Olive Oil is high in calories, so if you are trying to gain weight, add olive oil to all your meals!

Always use extra virgin expeller pressed, it's the highest quality available. The extra virgin is the first pressing of the flesh of the olive. (Regular olive oil is made from the pits and second pressings). My preference is Greek olive oil made from Kalama olives; it has a stronger flavor than Italian olive oil. When purchasing olive oil, always buy this product in a clear glass bottle in order to see the actual color of the oil; as usual, the richer and darker the oil, the better! Trader Joe's offers a non- organic 100% Greek Kalamata Extra Virgin Olive Oil.

Available: Trader Joe's

CHAPTER NINE

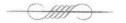

Condiments, Spices And Herbs... Oh My!

I Understand Why the Spice Trade Emerged; Food without Spices and Herbs is Like Life without Love—Rather Meaningless.

I have personally experienced all of the products in the following chapters. The recommendations are based on highest quality available and or best value / highest quality for the price, ease of use, and great taste!

Apple Sauce: Ideally, the applesauce label indicates the type of apples used; however, this is uncommon. Naturally, the only ingredient should be apples! So often it's a taste test that is required due to the lack of informative labeling.
Trader Joe's Organic Unsweetened Apple Sause has a great flavor.

Available: Trader Joe's

Basil: This herb is a wonderful addition to your Plant and Pray Garden. Basil contains trace minerals, is rich in vitamin K and flavonoid antioxidant compounds that protect the body's cells from free radical damage. They also contain volatile oils that hold antimicrobial and antibacterial properties. A study in the April 2011 issue of *Pharmaceutical Biology* reports that basil has antitumor properties and protects against chromosome damage caused by radiation treatments. Additionally, antihypertensive benefits, or the reduction of high blood pressure, are reported in the July 2010 issue of *Hypertension Research.*

There are also so many varieties of Basil! Some of my favorites include: Genovese Basil (the most common type), Greek Basil Lemon Basil, Thai Basil, Cinnamon Basil

Serving suggestions: Toss the basil leaves (and the flower buds from your Plant and Pray Garden) in your salads, or even substitute them for lettuce.

Bouillon:

Bouillon is an easy way to add additional flavor to rice and steamed or sautéed vegetables. When making soups also note that onions are naturally oily and are a common ingredient for soup stock and bouillon. When purchasing bouillon, choose one without preservatives, chemicals or added oils.

A delicious brand is Rapunzel Vegetable Bouillon with Herbs, a product of Switzerland.

Available: www.HealthyLivingWithDeirdre.com/Mark etplace & Whole Foods

Tip: Onions, which are naturally oily, are a common ingredient in soup stock and bouillon.

Catchup:

This is an American staple. Look for brands with no sugar or other extraneous ingredients. My favorite brand is Organic Ville, made with agave.

Available: www.HealthyLivingWithDeirdre.com/Mark etplace & Whole Foods

Chile Pepper:

Chile peppers contain capsaicin, the element that creates the heat or spiciness of a pepper. The Scoville scale is a measurement of the pungency (spicy heat) of chile peppers. By way of example, sweet bell peppers are 0 and some peppers can range to over 2,000! Many of the chile peppers my family enjoys are milder and in the 500 range. However, the more capsaicin, the better! Capsaicin has many healing properties; it helps to reduce pain and inflammation associated with arthritis, psoriasis, and diabetic neuropathy. Capsaicin also stops the spread of prostate cancer cells through a variety of mechanisms, (*Cancer Research*, March 15, 2016). It also stimulates secretions that help clear mucus from your system. As an extra plus: some research suggests that capsaicin can inhibit your desire for sweet and fatty foods.

Chile peppers also have insulin-lowering properties that can help control diabetes, according to a study published in the July 2006 issue of the *American Journal of Clinical Nutrition.*

Raw cacao chile peppers promote endorphin and serotonin release (The feel happy brain chemical), both of which inflate your mood.

Tip: By adding small amounts of chile peppers to your diet, you will slowly increase your tolerance to the spice and be able to consume more!

As a reminder, organic is always best because conventionally grown hot peppers are contaminated with concentrations of organophosphate insecticides, which are considered highly toxic to the nervous system.

Grow your own Chile peppers. Chile peppers are an excellent addition to the Plant and Pray Garden. When the first flowers appear, pick then off the plant; this promotes more flowers, and a more abundant crop. Also, when we discover critters excessively eating our vegetation, we apply cayenne pepper with water. Place the mixture in a spray bottle and spray the leaves. It is very effective and an environmentally responsible insecticide.

Some Some chile pepper varieties are available from Simply Organic in the form of a spice.

Cinnamon: Cinnamon, an ancient spice, offers a surprising number of health benefits. Cinnamon is one of the top seven anti-oxidants in the world, and it has both a wonderful calming aroma and a great taste! Many studies have found that anti-oxidants reduce the formation of free radicals that cause cancer.

Once again, brand and type do indeed matter when it comes to upgrading your health. There are two types of cinnamon.

Cassia cinnamon can be found in the grocery store.

Notes: (1) This type of cinnamon contains high levels of coumarin, which, when used in high dosages for extended periods of time can cause liver damage. (2) Coumarin (naturally occurring in some plants) is produced by the plant and works like a pesticide. Coumarin is responsible for the sweet smell of newly mowed hay.

Cassia cinnamon is most commonly consumed in North America, so beware of cinnamon as an ingredient in processed foods.

Another, far more **beneficial type** of cinnamon is **Ceylon cinnamon**. There are several professional studies concluding that cinnamon consumption reduces and helps to regulates blood sugars. It's also been used as part of a program for controlling weight and treating Type II diabetes. Kevin Gianni of RenegadeHealth.com states, "One animal study found that a particular component in cinnamon impaired the proliferation of cancer cells and slowed tumor growth." Ceylon cinnamon may also provide benefits to reducing risk of cancer, Alzheimer's, Parkinson's, and stomach problems, including gas and bloating associated with IBS, flu and much more. (Source: *Journal of Diabetes Science Technology*, May 1, 2010).

Cinnamaladehye, a component of cinnamon is a potent colorectal cancer fighter, as it starves the cancer cells of sugar.

Note: Ceylon cinnamon can also be used as a mosquito and black ant repellant, as a preservative, and as an odor neutralizer.

At my home, The Harbor Rose Bed & Breakfast, we use a variety of essential oils, including Ceylon cinnamon oil, to maintain a clean, eco-friendly environment for our guests to enjoy!

Brands for cinnamon sticks and ground powder include: Slimly Organic.

Available:
www.HealthyLivingWithDeirdre/com/Mark etplace, Whole Foods & Trader Joe's

Serving suggestion: Boil cinnamon stick to make tea as well as using the ground version when enjoying butternut squash or your morning oatmeal.

Brand for cinnamon oil:
The Ethica Company offers a single origin, wild crafted cinnamon oil.

Available:
www.HealthyLivingWithDeirdre.com/Mark etplace

Of Interest to Women:
Cinnamon has shown an amazing ability to stop medication-resistant yeast infections, including Escherichia coli bacteria and Candida Albicans fungus. Other studies suggest that its high levels of manganese are excellent for mitigating the effects of pre-menstrual syndrome (PMS).

Garlic:

Garlic contains antibacterial properties when consumed raw. Add some raw, finely chopped garlic to your soups and salads as a garnish. Store garlic on the counter in a basket that breathes, because the moisture from the fridge, or placing in a plastic bag will cause mold to form. My favorite variety of garlic has a purple hue to the clove skin; again, foods with purple are the "upgraded" option.

Garlic is a great item for the Plant and Pray Garden; the shoots are a lovely addition to salads. Remember, garlic is planted in the fall, as are other bulbs.

Hemp Seeds: These seeds are a great source of balanced omega fatty acids, which are very important for brain health. Hemp seeds are also high in protein. Three tablespoons of hemp seeds contain 10 grams of protein, along with iron, magnesium, zinc and phosphorus. Sprinkle on salads and steamed green beans, enjoy on fruit salad, and add to smoothies. They are also a very nice compliment to bananas.

The most tasty and fresh brand is Nutiva organic hemp seeds, raw and shelled.

Available: www.HealthyLivingWithDeirdre.com/Marketplace & Whole Foods

Mayo: Most American use a lot of mayonnaise. Traditionally, mayonnaise is made from eggs, and is therefore not vegan friendly. I have yet to find a person who can taste the difference between regular and grapeseed mayo, a much healthier option. This is an easy upgrade for you and your family.

My favorite brand is Follow your Heart Grapeseed Oil Vegenaise. Look for the one with the purple top as this company has a variety of options.

Available:
www.HealthyLivingWithDeirdre.com/Mark
etplace & Whole foods

Mustard: Many Americans are mustard fans. If you are one of them, I encourage you to try mustard greens as an upgrade when you are looking for that distinct mustard taste. My preference is Chinese mustard greens, as they have the qualities of delicate lettuce! Mustard greens or leaves of mustard plants are excellent source of essential minerals, including potassium calcium and phosphorous.

Try using mustard seeds in cooking. Mustard seeds are a rich source of minerals, including calcium, magnesium, phosphorous, selenium and potassium, which aid in weight loss and lowering cholesterol. Mustard seeds are also known to have anti-fungal and anti-bacterial properties. Indeed, mustard seeds are a good source of folate and vitamin A. Mustard seeds may also help control symptoms of asthma and have unique anti-inflammatory properties.

Mustard seeds
Simply Organic

Available:
www.HealthyLivingWithDeirdre.com/Mark
etplace & Whole Foods

Fresh mustard greens:
Available: Asian Markets

Mustard spread:
Westbrae Natural Organic Stoneground Mustard with no salt added is a tasty option.

Available:
www.HealthyLivingWithDeirdre.com/Mark etplace & Whole Foods

Oil of Oregano: This little ingredient is extremely important medicinally and very useful as a spice! Oil of oregano neutralizes fungus and mold spores, often found in fruit, but invisible to the naked eye. If you are eating fresh fruit, and especially berries, which are more prone to carrying molds and fungus, I highly recommend that you include three - to- five drops of oil of oregano in your meals the same day to mitigate this potential risk. When juicing vegetables, you can add three-to-four drops to a teaspoon of olive oil; the oregano flavor will permeate the juice. Add it to soup in the bowl, but do not cook it. Try adding a few drops to olive oil for your salad. It's especially delicious on pizza. Feel free to use it on any food that complements the strong flavor of oregano.

Oil of oregano can also be used on the gums to support gum health and reduce the risk of gingivitis. My daughter had a small spot of ringworm on her leg, caused by fungus or mold. Morning and evening treatments of a drop of oil of oregano on the skin cleared it right up in just a few days. I have also found that clients who suffer from reoccurring toe nail fungus and/or athletes foot experience absolute resolution of these issues once they add oil of oregano to their daily diet for an extended period of time.

My favorite brand is Natures Answer Alcohol-free Oil of Oregano, which can be found in the medicinal or supplement section of the market.

Available: www.HealthyLivingWithDeirdre.com/Mark etplace & Whole Foods

Olives:
Olives are a great source of healthy fats. Be sure to select olives that are packed in water and/or olive oil, and preferably extra virgin olive oil. Pitted Kalamata olives have a strong flavor; if you prefer a milder flavor, try pitted black olives.

Available: www.HealthyLivingWithDeirdre.com/Mark etplace & Trader Joe's

Parsley:
There is more calcium in an ounce of parsley than an ounce of milk. Parsley is rich in many vital vitamins, including vitamin C, B 12, K and A. This means parsley keeps your immune system strong, tones your bones and heals the nervous system. Parsley helps flush out excess fluid

from the body, thus supporting kidney function. Regular use of parsley can help control your blood pressure.

Use parsley any time you are seeking some green contrast to brighten up a dish.
I personally prefer Italian flat with larger leaves and stems; this type of parsley is especially delicious in salad and soup.

Peanuts &
Peanut Butter: Another American staple, peanuts are actually a manganese legume rather than a nut. Peanuts are a good source of vitamin E, niacin, folate, protein and manganese, high in antioxidants and feature brain and heart healthy benefits. The good news is that peanut butter is not very processed. According to the National Peanut Board, peanuts are the #1 snack nut in the US, accounting for two-thirds of all snack nuts consumed and an annual $2 billion. However, there are many concerns about consuming peanuts, one being that most commercial peanut butters are loaded with sugars and other food additives. What most people don't know is that when they enjoy America's favorite snack nut, they're likely ingesting mold and a toxic substance known as aflatoxins, a naturally occurring fungus / mold and a known carcinogen that has been linked to liver cancer. It is also highly possible that in some cases, peanut allergies are actually reactions to the mold rather than

the peanut itself. Aflatoxin is also known to stunt growth in children.

The liver is the body's filtration and detoxification system and must be maintained!

Higher amounts of mold are likely to be found in peanut butter as the lowest quality nuts are made into butters. Many are unaware that the FDA has very comprehensive requirements for all products consumed by humans. However, from my perspective, these quality standards leave much to be desired. The table below shows what levels of "non-peanut" substances are permitted in our peanut product food supply. The table below indicates the "Not to exceed the microbiological requirements dictated by the FDA." Translation: the FDA permitted levels of toxins in peanut products.

FDA Peanut Products Quality Standards:

Published May 2010

Microbiological Standards

Salmonella	**Negative**
E. Coli	**<3.6/g Most Probable Number (MPN)**
Coliform	**<10/g MPN**
Aerobic Plate Count	**<10,000/g**
Yeast	**<100/gram**
Mold	**<100/gram**
Aflatoxin	**<15 parts per billion (ppb)**

Organic is not necessarily any better, as aflatoxin is often still present. However, if you are a peanut lover there is a solution! The best tasting peanuts ever!

Raw Organic Wild Jungle Peanuts

These Amazon Rainforest wild peanuts are, unlike peanuts, free of mold and aflatoxins. This peanut, indigenous to Asia, has a unique appearance; it is mostly reddish with darker brown stripes. I shared some with a friend of mine who is an Oriental medicine doctor and holds a PHD in Herbalism. Her whole face lit up. "Where did you get these?" she asked. "I have not seen them for over 30 years! These are the peanuts we ate as children in China. I don't know what kind of peanuts they have here in the US, but they are not the peanuts I know and love!" Upgrading your diet is all about consuming the highest quality, less cultivated or "original food." If you like peanuts, you'll be pleasantly surprised by the delicious flavor of these wild peanuts. If you prefer peanut butter to whole peanuts, try making your own from these wild peanuts!

Wild Jungle Peanuts

Available: www.SunFood.Com

Pepper:

Regardless of the variety you prefer, freshly ground pepper is always best. Trader Joe's sells rainbow colored and black pepper in a self-grinding container.

Available: www.HealthyLivingWithDeirdre.com/Marketplace & Trader Joe's

Organic Grinder: 4 Seasons Pepper corns comes in a mill. Available: at Whole Foods

Pesto:

"Pesto" is Italian for anything ground up into a paste. If you are not making your own, look for ones made with olive oil. (My personal preference is pesto made from basil, pine nuts, garlic and olive oil.) Many companies do not tell you the type of basil used. Some companies add parsley and/or lower quality oils.

Serving suggestion: Try some on sandwiches, or as a dressing for quinoa, pasta or rice. A favorite in our house when homemade is not an option is Trader Giotto's Pesto Alla Genovese Basil Pesto. It's made with Genovese basil and extra virgin olive oil, and tastes great! It tastes great!

Available: www.HealthyLivingWithDeirdre.com/Marketplace and Trader Joe's

Note: Processed pesto often contains canola oil, so read the label carefully.

Pickles:

These are important fermented foods. However, vinegar should never be an ingredient, because fermentation or pickling process produces the flavor of vinegar. If the product already has vinegar as an ingredient, than you are not benefitting from the microbes that are produced in the pickling process. It is often difficult to find organic pickles. Enjoy the benefits of cucumbers plus the benefits of fermented foods that balance intestinal flora. My favorite brand is BA-TAMPTE, a kosher brand of half-sour pickles because they are fresh and crispy. All fresh pickles can be found in the refrigerated section. They have a short shelf life. Look for the very bright green ones that have just arrived and plan to consume them within a week. When they get too soft and the green loses its brightness, they are no longer crunchy. Naturally, all vegetables can be pickled, but cucumbers are the most commonly found pickles. Kimchee, a pickled cabbage that is a staple in the Korean diet, is worth a try. Traditional versions are very spicy; mild versions are also available.

Available: at local grocery stores and Whole foods. Also, try the Amish Farmer for some fresh pickles!

Pink Himalayan Sea Salt:

Table salt has aluminum chloride to reduce clumping: a known carcinogen. Sea salt is a better choice. However, sea salt is harvested from the ocean, and then washed and processed for packaging. Pink Himalayan sea salt is the best choice. Once you have tasted it, you will never return to your old salt! I even carry a small bit in my purse for when I'm eating out. If you find that clumping is an issue, just add a few grains of white rice to absorb the moisture. With 84 trace minerals, and hand mined, my favorite brand is The Original Himalayan Crystal Salt "Fine Granules."

Available:
www.HealthyLivingWithDeirdre.com/Mark etplace

Salsa: When making your selection, it's best to look for a brand with no added sugar, chemicals or canola oil. I have read a lot of salsa labels and I consistently find unacceptable ingredients. Amy's brand salsa contains nearly all organic ingredients and is made with filtered water. You guessed it! Organic salsa has a great flavor! The salsa comes in spicy, medium, and mild. I like to add fresh cilantro from my Plant and Pray Garden to freshen the salsa.

Available:
www.HealthyLivingWithDeirdre.com/Mark etplace &Whole Foods

Sauerkraut: Organic raw sauerkraut supports digestive flora. Again, avoid products with added vinegar or sugars and chemicals. You will find the best quality in the refrigerated section of the market. My favorite is Deep

Root—it's raw, organic and sold in a bag in the refrigerated section.

Available: Whole Foods

Sour Cream: Like all other dairy products, sour cream should always be organic and used in moderation. My favorite is Trader Joe's Organic Sour Cream; it has a very nice flavor and is not bitter like many other organic sour cream brands. Another good source for sour cream is your local Amish farmer.

Available: Trader Joe's & Amish Farmer

Soy Sauce: Soy sauce is actually made from fermented soybeans aged in oak casks, much the way wine is. When making a selection, confirm there are no hidden sugars or chemical ingredients. For those who have celiac disease or wheat sensitivity, soy sauce is also available in a gluten free form called Tamari, a more concentrated form of soy sauce. Tamari can also be used as an egg replacement when frying something breaded, such as eggplant; it makes the breadcrumbs stick like an egg does.

My favorite soy sauce is Ohsawa Organic Nama Shoyu. Given the varying quality of soy sauce, when visiting your local Japanese restaurant, you might choose, as I do, to bring your own!

Available:
www.HealthyLivingWithDeirdre.com/Mark
etplace & Whole foods

Tahini: Tahini made from dark sesame seeds is much more nutritious and tasty than is Tahini made from white sesame. As a rule, always use the more colorful (or darker) version of an ingredient when available. My preference is raw organic black sesame tahini, served on pasta, rice, or as a snack. It's especially tasty spread on banana.
My favorite brand is Artisana.

Available:
www.HealthyLivingWithDeirdre.com/Mark
etplace

**Sundried
Tomatoes:**   It's best to buy sundried tomatoes packed in olive oil or no oil at all. I prefer the julienne sliced; they are handy to put on sandwiches or to top a pizza. My favorite is Trader Joe's brand Julienne Sliced Sun-dried Tomatoes, available in a small jar.

Available at Trader Joe's

Turmeric Root: Can be found fresh at Whole Foods when in season, and is most often found in powder form. This root, which is ground and comes in the form of a spice, is a powerful curative that has long been used in Chinese and Indian medicine as an anti-inflammatory agent to treat a wide variety of conditions.

Sprinkle it into soups or on mashed potatoes. Frontier brand is a good choice because it is tasty, organic, and easy to find. That said, I find that the freshest brand is Wild Harvest.

Available:
www.HealthyLivingWithDeirdre/com/Mark etplace & Whole Foods

Vinegar:

If you are not a fan of vinegar, it may be because you have not enjoyed high quality vinegar. High quality vinegar creates instant salad fans!

Traditionally made from grapes, vinegar's antioxidant properties fight cancer, reduce risk of heart attack, control diabetes, assist in digestion and stabilize cholesterol levels.

The infused flavors are endless. Some of my favorite balsamic vinegars are apple, dark chocolate, fig and cinnamon pear. There are also white vinegars that are quite tasty, including oregano and peach vinegars, which have a very bright flavor.

Two gourmet imported olive oil and vinegar shops include Olive Tree, and the Crushed Olive, both of which ship anywhere in the US.

www.OliveTreeLongIsland.com
www.TheCrushedOlive.com

CHAPTER TEN

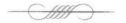

Prepared Foods... *In Case Of Emergency!*

Snacks and prepared foods are often alluring, with their high sugar and salt content. Once more, be careful about reading labels. Some of these products have health-damaging ingredients. Beware of aluminum, dyes, hidden dairy, sugars, soy, and any of the other 10,000 food additives and other chemicals that have been approved by the FDA. Favor higher quality oils such as coconut oil and olive oil. Safflower and sunflower oils are of lesser quality, but acceptable so long as they are GMO free. If a product contains the amorphous label "vegetable oil," I run the other way, because I don't know what I'm getting. Finally, omit nonorganic wheat and other ingredients you don't recognize. Also, be aware of products with a high sugar, dairy, or soy content.

Tomato Sauce: The best tasting tomato sauce is organic and made from fresh tomatoes. This is also the most expensive. You want to look for tomato sauce with no oil and no sugar because you can always add your own high quality oil and sweeteners. My favorites include Rao's Homemade Marinara (spicy), Arrabbiata

Available: Whole Foods

Uncle Steve's Organic Tomato & Basil, Uncle Steve's Organic Arrabbiata (nicely spiced), Uncle Steve's Organic Marinara, Available: Whole Foods

Burgers: If you find you have a taste for meat, try buffalo burgers. They are not produced in factory farms like beef. They are always grass fed, and the meat contains less fat and fewer calories than beef. Buffalo meat also has a stronger, more "meaty" taste, which many meat eaters find more satisfying. This often results in their eating less meat. If you want to try veggie burgers, it's best to avoid soy, sugars and, of course, canola oil! I have found two vegetable burger companies that I recommend. For current veggie burger fans, I recommend Organic Sunshine Burgers; the Southwest version is especially tasty. I fry them in organic, unflavored coconut oil and serve them over a bed of Herb Blend Baby Field Greens, with some friend onions and mushrooms. Add pickles, catchup and enjoy!

If you're looking for a meaty-tasting substitute, try Field Roast Burgers. They are delicious and have the texture of real meat, without any of the downsides. This company offers many other products, all of which are very tasty.

Organic Sunshine Burgers South West
Available: Whole Foods – Frozen
Field Roast Burgers: Whole Foods –Frozen

While the development of cancer is influenced by both environment and genetic factors, there is also a body of evidence that consumption of animal proteins is each linked to a particular form of cancer is best evidenced in the book, *The China Study* authored by T. Colin Campbell (a former dairy farmer) and Thomas M Campbell MD. This study is considered by many to be the most comprehensive study of nutrition ever conducted. The book has startling implications for diet, weight loss, and long-term health.

It is the culmination of a 40-year research study with the participation of several universities. In short, the researchers concluded that the type of animal protein consumed determines the type of cancer and / or other debilitating diseases humans develop. Eat plants and live longer and healthier lives. Naturally, any powerful study that gets a lot of press also attracts some "push back," as has the China Study. Some people are seeking to discredit the findings. I will speak more about my opinions on the subject of studies later in the book. I believe what is ultimately most valuable is doing your own research in order to experience how different foods affect you!

Interested in learning more about plant-based diets vs meat and dairy diets? Do you prefer movies? You may enjoy documentaries such as: "Forks over Knives," "Food Matters," "Food Inc.," "Fat, Sick and Nearly Dead," and "Super-Size Me." This documentary resulted in the new product "apple fries" now available at McDonalds.

Field Roast Sausages: Artesian and Vegan Field Roast Sausages are also a delicious meat alternative. A traditional Italian dish (and one of my favorites) is sausage and peppers with onions, typically served with tomato sauce on a hero. I have often made this dish with the Field Roast Sausages and people LOVE them, and believe it is real Italian meat sausage. While my personal favorite flavor is Italian, all the flavors are worth a try! If you like breakfast sausages, this brand is a delicious option.

Available: Whole Foods

Frozen Prepared Foods

When shopping for frozen prepared foods, the emphasis, once again, is on products that contain real ingredients. Locate products that do not contain hidden dairy, soy or sugars, canola oil, salt, food additives or chemicals. If baking powder is an ingredient, it should be "aluminum free" baking powder. Unfortunately, not many frozen foods meet these criteria.

My family chooses not to eat corn as a side vegetable due to its high glycemic load. However, a sprinkle of bright yellow can be a fun addition to black rice and black bean salsa. Try a few tablespoons in a vegetable soup or even an arugula salad. Bright, sweet, yellow corn has a festive visual effect while adding a touch of sweetness to any dish. Organic super sweet corn is absolutely and undeniably delicious.

Available: Traders Joe's – Frozen

Corn Meal Crust Pizza Shells: This product is tasty and has good, non-GMO ingredients. The crust stays nice and crunchy. This is also a deep-dish version, so you can fill it with your favorite toppings. In my experience, Whole Foods does not always stock this ingredient, so be sure to ask before making a separate trip.

Available: Whole Foods frozen section

Vicollapizza.com

Falafels: Falafels are a Middle Eastern / Mediterranean favorite, traditionally packed with nutritious parsley. They are nice to have on hand and are an easy way to get beans/ legumes into the diet of the "non-bean" friendly folks. Enjoy them in some tahini or slide them into a cucumber sandwich. If you don't have time to make your own, try a non-organic frozen option that is not all bad.

Cooking tip: Fry them for about five minutes in unflavored coconut oil until golden brown

Brand: Falafelim frozen uncooked Falafel balls. Available: Whole Foods

Frozen Fruit: This is a staple in our home. We defrost a bowl and enjoy a taste of summer all year long. Try adding berries to smoothies or serve them over buckwheat pancakes.

Some of my favorite brands include:
Organic Mixed Berry Blend
Available: Trader Joe's

Organic Wild Blueberries
Available: Trader Joe's

Organic Strawberries
Available: Trader Joe's

Peppers: Fresh and organic is always best, although a bag of frozen peppers can be helpful in a pinch when making a quick batch of chili.

Mélange a Troas is a non-organic frozen option.

Available: Trader Joe's

Pizza: Amy's Corn Meal Crust 3 Cheese Pizza is my favorite, since this product combines vegetables with protein / dairy rather than a grain like rice or wheat, making it the highest profit frozen pizza I have found. I always keep one in my freezer; it's easy for a quick play date snack and most kids love pizza! Why not introduce a high quality option to the neighborhood kids?

Available: Whole Foods

Chips, Nuts and Other Salty Crunchy Snacks
Banana Chips: This is a great snack that contains higher quality oils, such as safflower or sunflower. It's not easy to find this organic, but you might try your local organic markets. Roasted Plantain Chips are a nonorganic option.

Available: Trader Joe's

Corn Chips: Corn is one of the foods we need to be super careful about. A full eighty per cent of the US corn supply is genetically engineered with pesticide spliced directly into the DNA. As the monarch butterfly population migrates across the Great Plains, some experts say that approximately 50% of them die from eating corn along the way. When you choose to eat corn, eat organic. Also, be sure there is high quality oil as an ingredient. Try… Organic Blue Corn Chips; lose the guilt and get the benefits of blue/purple food! My favorite brands include Trader Joe's Organic Corn Chip Dippers (yellow).

Available: Trader Joe's

Organic Blue Corn Chip:

Simply Sprouted: Way Better Snacks – Simply Unbeatable Blues Corn Tortilla Chips (I find these are a bit on the salty side and lovely for guacamole.)

Available www.HealthyLivingWithDeirdre.com/Marketplace & Whole Foods

Full Circle – Organic Blue Corn Tortilla Chips

Available: Whole Foods

Kamut Cakes:

These cakes have a higher nutritional value than rice cakes. I like kamut cakes for times when I'm not really hungry, but feel like chewing something. At 20 calories a cake, they are crunchy and do the trick. Note: If you chew as long as possible before swallowing, you will taste the simple sugars.

My favorite brand is Susie's Whole Ancient Grain Kamut Puffed Cakes Lightly Salted.

Available:
www.HealthyLivingWithDeirdre.com/Mark etplace & Whole Foods

Nuts: Always purchase raw and organic nuts for their nutritional value and taste. Raw nuts don't have added oils or salt. I also recommend eating more nuts in harmony with the winter season, because they are freshest then. Before consuming nuts, always soak them in purified alkaline water overnight. Soaking activates the life force in the nuts, and also softens the nuts, making them easier to chew and digest. Fresh whole raw nuts when sprouted should grow into a tree. These are the highest quality nuts. Nuts that are not broken or processed in any way.

Available: Trader Joe's & Whole Foods

Popcorn: Use organic popcorn and enjoy the ease of popping your own. Preparation: In a pot with a cover, place a layer of organic corn kernels, add Organic Gold Label Coconut Oil to cover the kernels, and pop on a medium low heat. Add pink Himalayan sea salt and grated sheep milk cheese and serve. (I have yet to find a prepackaged brand that I would recommend.)

Potato Chips: When choosing potato chips look for those with sea salt; ideally, the type of the potato and type of oil—sunflower and safflower oils are the highest grade available—will be listed on the package. I find that salt and pepper chips are best, as it's harder to eat too many! My favorite brand is Kettle Brand Organic Salt & Pepper chips.

Available: Whole Foods

Seaweed: When we eat processed food or restaurant food, we often balance it with seaweed in the same meal, thereby replacing the minerals that were removed in the refining process. As my grandfather said, "It's all going to the same place and all the parts should arrive together!" If you are constantly thinking out loud about balancing your meals, glycemic load, and minerals with high color content foods, your children will begin thinking that way too. When my daughter was three years old, we went to the beach. She was playing in the shallow water of the bay, stomping her feet and running in and out of the water when a piece of seaweed caught her ankle. She picked it up and yelled "Mommy, look! The ocean wants to feed me. Can I eat it?" She recognizes food everywhere!

When making seaweed selections, it is often difficult to find brands that do not contain canola oil—also called rapeseed oil—and/or added sugars. For snacking, the roasted single servings are a good option. The Love brand is the best option I have found. The downside is that it is roasted with olive oil, which is good oil; however, roasting at high temperatures creates free radicals. On the plus side, it is non-GMO Verified and chemical free.

Available:
www.HealthyLivingWithDeirdre.com/Mark etplace

For my daughter's birthday party at the beach, we included the single serve seaweed snacks for the children. I remember a friend asking me, "What child is going to eat seaweed at a birthday party?" The answer was all of them! Children love the individually wrapped snacks and the salty flavor provided by the minerals. Many parents were surprised when their children asked for more!

CHAPTER ELEVEN

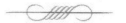

I Want Something Sweet:
Desserts, Ice Cream And Sweeteners!

**Candy Bars &
Energy Bars:**   There are so many delicious and organic fruit, nut and energy bars without added sugar, dairy or soy that can serve as a very satisfying replacement for candy bars. When I traveled 180 days a year, I always kept several Greens Plus Energy Bars on hand in case a real meal was not available.

Greens Plus Energy Bars
Chocolate Greens Plus Energy Bars

Available:
www.HealthyLivingWithDeirdre/com/Mark etplace, Trader Joe's & Whole Foods

Keep Healthy – New York State Bar
Cashew Date Bar & Pecan Bar

Available:
www.HealthyLivingWithDeirdre.com/Mark etplace

Chocolate: There is a long romantic history between humans and chocolate, also known as cacao.

Chocolate contains dopamine, which is a natural painkiller. Serotonin, which is also found in chocolate, produces feelings of pleasure. Even the smell of chocolate causes relaxation; it significantly reduces theta activity in the brain, associated with attention, and relaxing the subject. (Source: *International Journal of Psychophysiology*, 1998).

When we were teenagers, a chocolate bar served as currency for solving many problems, including peacemaking, consolation (especially after doing poorly on a test), and surviving heartbreak. Somehow, chocolate makes everything better! And there is additional scientific research to support this emotional improvement! Cacao, the bean that chocolate is made from, also boosts brain levels of serotonin, the "feel good" brain chemical. But it does far more than that! Cacao contains over 700 complex antioxidants known as polyphenols, which help reduce 'bad cholesterol. Raw cacao also balances hormones, and the flavanols (also found in green tea and dark-colored fruits), are heart-healthy and anti-inflammatory, possibly protecting against cardiovascular disease.

Chocolate contains over 300 chemicals, including a multitude of vitamins, minerals (calcium, iron, potassium, magnesium).

Fall in love with divine: chocolate contains a chemical called phenyl ethylamine, which is released naturally in the body when you fall in love and is also considered an aphrodisiac.

However, consumer be warned! If in the process of making chocolate, the temperature rises over 120 degrees, many of the nutritional benefits are lost. The most typical "Dutch Process" results in a darker color and nutrient loss. The preferred process, or raw cacao, results in a lighter color and more nutrients for your body to enjoy. Try a tablespoon or two of raw cacao mixed with a cup of warm coconut milk before meals if you want to lose weight. Cacao is a natural MAO inhibitor: it shrinks the appetite.

Did you know? The Department of Nutrition at University of California, Davis discovered that cacao thins blood and can even prevent blood clots!

If you are eating commercial grade (Mars or Hershey type) milk chocolate bars, upgrade to a higher quality dark chocolate and try organic brands like Green and Black (85% cacao—no soy lecithin—is a bonus!). Here's why: when cacao is mixed with dairy, the dairy blocks the body's ability to absorb the beneficial antioxidants. If you are ready to benefit from the healing nutritional of chocolate, stick with the raw and less-processed versions.

Tip: Always choose a brand that is organic, unsweetened, and has no other ingredients. You can always add high quality sweeteners.

Trader Joe's has a good tasting, non-organic option that is an upgrade from commercial baker's chocolate, but not as nutritious as the versions available from: Logenvity-warehouse.com.

Available: Trader Joe's

Organic Raw 100% Arriba Criollo Cacao Powder, among many other high quality chocolate products.

Available: www.LongevityWarehouse.com

Other favorite options include:
Cacao Nibs: Try mixing them with raisins

Available:
www.HealthyLivingWithDeirdre.com/Marketplace

Navitas Cacao Powder is a preferred powdered choice.

Available:
www.HealthyLivingWithDeirdre.com/Marketplace & Whole Foods

Sunfood Cacao Nips and Powder

Available:
www.HealthyLivingWithDeirdre.com/Mark etplace & SunFood.com

Alter Eco Chocolate Bars and Truffles (soy lecithin free)

Available:
www.HealthyLivingWithDeirdre.com/Mark etplace & Whole Foods

Living Raw Truffles that come in a variety of flavors.

Available:
www.HealthyLivingWithDeirdre.com/Mark etplace

Lily's Chocolate (The soy lecithin in Lily's is organic, and is non-GMO and hexane-free) but I'd prefer soy free).

Available:
www.HealthyLivingWithDeirdre.com/Mark etplace

It is important to note that even if chocolate, or another item, is labeled organic that does not always translate into "safe to consume."

Here is a quote from As You Sow: "Responding to published research showing high levels of heavy metals in commonly eaten food items, As You Sow began extensive independent laboratory testing of 42 chocolate products for lead and cadmium. We found that 26 of the chocolate products (62%) contain lead and/or cadmium at levels in which one serving exceeds the California safe harbor level for reproductive harm. We filed notices with 16 manufacturers, including Mars, Hershey, Lindt, Godiva, Whole Foods, and others, for failing to provide required warnings to consumers that their chocolate products contain lead, cadmium, or both." For more information visit http://www.asyousow.org/our-work/environmental-health/toxic-enforcement/lead-and-cadmium-in-food/

Note: No level of lead is safe for children!

Cookies:

When it comes to cookies, sometimes you just have to have one! It's nearly impossible to find a commercial cookie without sugar, but thanks to Pamela's, there are some fantastic gluten- and dairy-free options. My favorites are Pamela's Chunky Chocolate Chip and Pamela's Pecan Shortbreads.

Available: www.HealthyLivingWithDeirdre.com/Mark etplace & Whole Foods

Fruit Roll Ups:

When choosing, always seek a brand with no added sugars and no ingredients other than fruit. Again, European brands are safer, as they don't have GMO ingredients. A new brand we recently discovered is made in Belgium; the brand is N.A. Nature Addicts Fruit Sticks. (www.na-natureaddicts.com). We tried the Apple Raspberry and it is quite tasty.

Available: www.HealthyLivingWithDeirdre.com/Mark etplace

Ice Cream & Ice Pops:

These are, of course, a favorite on hot summer days. There are now several companies that offer nondairy options for these cooling treats.

Below are some of my favorites:
Coconut Bliss and Naked Coconut, both coconut-based desserts, sweetened with agave. Both coconut milk and coconut cream are high in good quality fats.

Also worth a try is Coconut Bliss Organic Mint Galactica, which comes in a one-pint container, making portion control easier. It is also sweetened with agave. It's delicious, and my clear favorite!

Serving tip: This product is creamier and more flavorful it you leave it on the counter for 10 minutes or so, before serving.

Available: Whole Foods

Eat POPs Green Detox, a green juice frozen treat, is a favorite in my household! There are many other Eat POPs flavors worth exploring.

A rich and creamy favorite of mine is So Delicious Coconut Milk Fudge Pops – sweetened with agave.

Available: Whole Foods

Sweeteners

Date Syrup:

Date syrup is a new and deliciously sweet addition to the pantry. The massive health benefits of dates have made them one of the best ingredients for muscle development; they're especially effective for marathon runners to nibble on as they race. Dates are packed with nutrients, vitamins, fiber, iron and calcium. Benefits of dates include relief from constipation, intestinal disorders, heart problems, anemia, sexual dysfunction, diarrhea, abdominal cancer, and many other conditions. Enjoy a date each day. If you are seeking to gain weight, add a few more.
My favorite brand of date syrup is
Date Lady Pure Date Syrup; it's organic and has only one ingredient—organic dates!

Available:
www.HealthyLivingWithDeirdre.com/Mark etplace & Whole Foods

Honey: There are many healing properties associated with honey, which contains a variety of vitamins and minerals, and is known to boost athletic performance. The type of vitamins and minerals and their quantity depends on the type of flowers used for apiculture. Its exact balance of fructose and glucose actually helps the body regulate blood sugar levels. Honey also contains flavonoid antioxidants which help reduce the risk of some cancers and heart disease. Recent research shows that honey treatments may help disorders such as ulcers and bacterial gastroenteritis. Honey has anti-bacterial and anti-fungal properties as well.

"All honey is antibacterial, because the bees add an enzyme that makes hydrogen peroxide," said Peter Molan, director of the Honey Research Unit at the University of Waikato in New Zealand. Manuka honey is, made in New Zealand from the nectar of leptospermum scoparium (New Zealand tea tree), which is sometimes used to treat chronic leg ulcers and pressure sores. It's the basis of Med Honey, a leading line of medical grade honey products used for burns and wounds. Manuka honey is also largely made from the pollen of the tea tree blossom, a blossom known for its antibacterial properties.

Honey is tried and true, as it has been used for 4,000 years in Ayurveda medicine in

India. It is considered to positively affect all three of the body's primitive material imbalances. It is also said to be useful in improving eyesight, weight loss, curing impotence and premature ejaculation, urinary tract disorders, bronchial asthma, diarrhea, and nausea.

It is also important to remember that honey is not safe for children under one year old because their immune system is not amply developed to fight the botulism spores that might make their way into the honey.

It is also important to note that the healing benefits of honey are contained in raw unfiltered honey that is not heated above 180 degrees. More common cooked commercial grade honey can be as bad as white sugar. Also, be mindful that if you have pollen allergies, it might be best not to consume honey until those allergies are cleared.

When honey is consumed with warm water, it helps in digesting the fat stored in your body.

Serving suggestion: Enjoy a bit of honey in warm water, add some cinnamon and lemon juice, and enjoy a delightful weight-loss soothing beverage.

As always, it is best to know your food source; most areas have beekeeper associations who are always a good source of local honey.

When purchasing Manuka honey there is a variety of choices available from Manuka Health.

Available:
www.HealthyLivingWithDeirdre.com/Mark etplace

Note: MGO certified indicated the product has been tested by independent laboratories.

Maple Syrup: Besides being delicious, maple syrup is anti-inflammatory, antioxidant rich, immune system-boosting, and heart-healthy maintaining. It also aids in male reproductive health. When making a selection, organic and less processed is best, the darker the color the better. When available, it's also best to buy local. Explore and add this important sweetener to your daily living experience.

Available:
www.HealthyLivingWithDeirdre/com/Mark etplace, Trader Joe's & Whole Foods

Raw Blue Agave: When buying raw blue agave, look for the darker, less-processed color. You'll be able to see the color better if you buy the product in a clear container. Remember to combine with high fiber and/or high fat content foods, such as yams, coconut milk and/or coconut cream. Use sparingly. It is very sweet and goes a long way. As always, seek agave that is both organic and raw.

Available: Trader Joe's

CHAPTER TWELVE

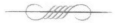

Let's Drink To Good Health!...
Beverages, Coffee, Tea, Milk, Soda, Water

Almond Milk: This milk is a good replacement for beverage creamers. Remember that this is produced from a nut, so it's best not to mix with grains and cereal. For milk replacement combined with cereal, try coconut milk. I recommend Almond Breeze brand: unsweetened.

Available: www.HealthyLivingWithDeirdre.com/Marketplace & Whole Foods

Coffee: Drink less, and select fair trade organic. Fair trade coffee is coffee that is certified as having been produced by fair trade standards. Not-for-profit fair trade organizations create trading partnerships based on dialogue, transparency and respect that seeks greater equity in international trade. Fair Trade is a voluntary program utilized by coffee importers and food companies to create an alternative market for traditionally disadvantaged producers in developing countries, usually small-scale farmers. Kona coffee from Hawaii is the least acidic, and therefore, one of the best commercial coffee choices commonly available. If you are consuming caffeinated coffee, and you'd like to wean yourself from caffeine, take these simple steps that worked for me. With each cup of coffee add a splash of decaf. Continue to add a larger splash until you are drinking decaf with a splash of regular coffee. This process will gradually help to avoid the headaches that often come with caffeine withdrawal. Once you have moved to decaf only coffee, you may want to move to the next step. Try INKA brand instant grain beverage. It's a power of only good ingredients and has a similar smell and flavor to that of coffee. It's quite satisfying.

Note: Caffeine causes one to crave sweets. If you are a person who struggles with sugar cravings, eliminating caffeine from your diet will make it a lot easier to eliminate refined sugars and feel those cravings for sweets disappear!

Available:
www.HealthyLivingWithDeirdre.com/Mark etplace

Longevity Warehouse now features Artisan high quality coffee in a variety of different roasts. This brand is certified organic, tested to be 100% free of all mycotoxins and fungus by-products," (common in organic coffee beans). It also has a pH of 7.2, the

ideal pH for our alkaline-loving bodies!).
Note: Contains caffeine.

Available: www.LongevityWarehouse.com

Soda: Carbonated beverages cause extreme acidity, partly due to the sugars and mostly created by the carbonation. Never consume diet soda. If you are hooked on cola, wean yourself off by trying Tianfu China Cola, its caffeine-free, GMO-free, and a better alternative to the more commercial brands.

Available: Whole Foods

Tea: Tea is simply any plant boiled in water. Reduce your consumption of caffeine by trying some non-caffeinated herbal teas. Try making your own tea with herbs from your Plant and Pray Garden. Toss any herbs or spices into your alkaline water and boil. Look for naturally caffeine-free teas. Try a cinnamon stick in boiling water; it's quite tasty. My favorite tea brands include: Yogi and Traditional Medicinals.

Available:
www.HealthyLivingWithDeirdre.com/Mark
etplace & Whole Foods

Green Tea: This ancient beverage has powerful medicinal properties and an abundance of nutrients, minerals and powerful antioxidants that protect cells from damage. Green tea also contains L-theanine, which increases the activity of the inhibitory neurotransmitter GABA, which has anti-anxiety effects. It also increases dopamine. The production of alpha waves in the brain, when combined with the trace amounts of caffeine found in green tea, improves brain function. Some studies show that green tea increases the metabolism and burns fat. Green tea reduces the risk of many cancers, including breast, prostate and colorectal cancer. Many studies conclude that green tea also protects your brain as we age, potentially lowering the risk of Alzheimer's and Parkinson's. It may also inhibit the growth of bacteria and some viruses and improve dental health. And if that is not enough, some studies show it also reduces the risk of Type II diabetes by improving insulin sensitivity and reducing sugar levels. Green tea has been shown to lower total and LDL cholesterol, as well as protecting the LDL particles from oxidation. It is also very effective in reducing dangerous abdominal fat. Another study in 14,001 elderly Japanese individuals aged 65-84 years found that those who consumed the most green tea were 76% less likely to die during the six-year study period. Other studies have shown greater longevity among those enjoying green tea daily.

Green Tea Extract inhibits the storage of excess carbohydrates as body fat and preferentially diverts them to muscle cells.

I drink between 3 to 5 liters of green tea daily. Each day I prepare five (5) liter thermoses and take them everywhere, and there is always enough to share! I drink a very high quality and use the leaves for multiple infusions so the tea is very light, nearly hot water with a suggestion of tea. My favorite green tea is Oolong Tie Kuan Yin Iron Goddess of Mercy, which originated in Fujian province China. Like wine, teas have annual competitions, and I prefer the higher grade early spring leaves, which are often handpicked and monkey rolled (loose tea). Tea bags typically have the lowest quality leaves, or crumbs of what once were leaves.

Tip: When traveling extensively, and if you're choosy about your tea, try travelling with Chi Tea Green Tea extract. Simply put 20 drops or so in hot alkaline water and it's all good! It contains 95% green tea and has the added benefit of other medicinal herbs. If you have loved ones who are working to increase their water intake and they are seeking additional flavor, add this green tea extract.

Chi Tea Green Tea Extract
Available:
www.HealthyLivingWithDeirdre.com/Marketplace

Iron Goddess Tea Leaves: When making a selection, look for Tie Kuan Yin Iron

Goddess of Mercy organic, spring tea leaves that are handpicked from Fujian province China.

I have tried some sources from www.aliexpress.com with some success, although the site is a bit difficult to navigate.

Milk: Cow and other animal milk is food for baby animals; many experts agree that nature did not design animal milk for human consumption. However, if you're a dedicated milk drinker, try raw, un-pasteurized un-homogenized organic goat milk.

Available: Amish Farmer

Coconut Milk: Coconut milk is the best choice when mixing with grains. Be sure when making a selection that there are no added sweeteners or other ingredients. You will find two options: regular full fat coconut milk and light coconut milk. Coconut fat is a great, healthy fat. However, if you are consuming other healthy fats you may want to try the light version. Use coconut milk to replace dairy when baking and / or when preparing "cream of" soups and mashed potatoes. You might also try it in your cereal.

My favorite brands are Thai Kitchen Organic (Thai Kitchen also has a non-organic version) and Native Forest.

Available:
www.HealthyLivingWithDeirdre.com/Mark
etplace & Whole Foods

Coconut Water: This is nature's perfect food. If you find yourself dehydrated, you can actually put coconut water straight into your veins through an IV. That's right; it is compatible with human blood plasma! Did you know that coconut water has an abundance of electrolytes? Coconut water lowers blood pressure, nourishes skin, aids in digestion and weight loss and clears up blemishes. Disregard those other sports drinks, and switch to raw organic coconut water. (It's also the ultimate hangover remedy and is very useful if you or your kids have been sick and vomiting, as it's full of electrolytes.) When making a selection, look for only one ingredient: organic coconut water.

My favorite brand is Harmless Harvest Coconut Water. It comes in a BPA-free bottle, and it's USDA organic. Sometimes the liquid is pink rather than clear; this is simply evidence of the naturally varying antioxidants in the coconut water.

Available:
www.HealthyLivingWithDeirdre.com/Mark
etplace & Whole Foods

Coconut Cream: This cream is so very rich and serves as a nutritious alternative to whipped cream. It provides an excellent source of healthy fat. Be mindful that it will begin to melt at over 72 degrees. When using it as whip cream, put the can in the fridge for an hour or so, and be sure it stays upright. Open it, and drain out the excess liquid. Place a stainless steel bowl in the freezer for one hour and place the coconut cream in the cold bowl. Add a bit of vanilla and a dash of maple syrup, date syrup, or agave. Use an electric mixer to whip for just a minute or so to whip the ingredients together, and enjoy your dairy-free delicious topping with berries or on a cupcake. Native Forest has an organic version.

Available: www.HealthyLivingWithDeirdre.com/Marketplace

Trader Joe's has a non-organic version that is not all that bad.

Available: Trader Joe's

Water: We've already mentioned that it's best to store or carry water in glass containers or stainless steel water bottles. We never leave the house without a stainless steel thermos! Make your own alkaline water, or purchase water from a place like Phountain. Drink and cook with alkaline water. If you prefer to flavor your water, add freshly squeezed lemon or lime. If the mood suits you, or just for fun, add a dash of maple or date syrup!

CHAPTER THIRTEEN

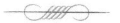

Grains & Breads, Beans, Legumes And Pasta

Bread

Generally speaking, minimize bread and pasta and increase whole grains, beans and legumes. Our family consumes two servings per person of pasta a week, and only one slice of bread per person per week. We consider these food options to be high quality "junk food," so we always balance them with plenty of no-glycemic load alkalizing vegetables and/or seaweed.

Hearty Breads

Ezekiel 4:9

When making a bread selection, follow the same rule as when selecting other foods: look for good oils and no added sugars or chemicals. As always, watch out for unrecognizable ingredients and/or preservatives. Remember, the fewer ingredients a product has, the better! Bread is made from flour, so it's best not to consume too much. Why, you ask? When a grain is pulverized into flour, this increases the glycemic load. By increasing the glycemic load, you are reducing the fuel or energy that the grain offers in its whole state, before it became flour. Flour is yet another processed food. High profit foods are synonymous with less processing.

That said, some flour products are healthier than others. Ezekiel 4:9 is a favorite of mine, and the company offers a variety of flavors and shapes. All are sprouted and come in loaves. Consider trying the cinnamon raisin English muffins- great with and bilberry jam and goat butter! These breads freeze well and are often found in the freezer section in your local organic market.

Available: Whole Foods and Trader Joe's

Tip: The best way to preserve bread is to freeze it.

Millet Bread:

The brand I recommend is a great replacement for white bread and is also ideal for making breadcrumbs! This bread is great toasted and works very well for bruschetta and pizza, as it will not get soggy for many hours. The Deland Bakery brand recipe uses filtered water and brown rice flour as well as millet. This tasty treat comes in many different shapes and sizes, including hot dog and hamburger rolls, bagels, regular loaves and large flat rounds that I like to use for bruschetta and pizza. Some local artisan markets carry this brand. I called the bakery to find a local market nearby that carried their products.

Available: www.DelandBakery.com.

Call the bakery and ask them what markets in your area carry their products. You will notice there are few breads made with purified water.

Muffins: Organic Moral Fiber Blueberry Bran Muffins are a nice treat once in a while. I like them sliced and lightly toasted with a bit of cambozola cheese. This is a "no no" food combination that I treat myself to once or twice a year; I have also found these muffins to be useful as "pretend cupcakes" when my daughter attends a birthday party. At times, I'll bring this treat for her as a replacement for traditional cupcakes served at the party.

Available: Trader Joe's

Tortillas: Tortillas are usually made from corn; we have to be mindful when we select corn that 100% of the ingredients are organic and not GMO. Also, purchase tortillas with higher quality oils, such as sunflower or safflower oils. The highest quality tortillas will include sprouted grains, since sprouting activates the life force in the grains.

Ezekiel 4:9 sprouted grain tortillas are based on the biblical recipe. This is a great option for quesadillas.

Available:
www.HealthyLivingWithDeirdre.com/Mark etplace & Whole foods

Oatmeal: Commonly referred to as America's healthiest breakfast food! It's already well publicized that oatmeal reduces bad cholesterol and maintains heart health. I highly recommend substituting organic steal cut oats for the more traditional oatmeal. Organic steal cut oats have the lowest glycemic load, and therefore deliver long-burning fuel, as the oats are in a less processed state. And as always when making a selection, be sure there are no added sugars and avoid instant anything! When you prepare it yourself you can ensure that high quality alkaline water was used.

Organic Steel Cut Oats

Available: Trader Joe's

Pasta: In order to make our pasta more nourishing, we make a pasta sauce with lots of veggies, including onions and peppers, herbs, and olives and add extra virgin olive oil to each plate when serving.

My favorites are quinoa pasta & brown rice pasta. It's best to enjoy the quinoa pasta al dente; if overcooked, it gets very sticky and can become like mush.

Ancient Harvest Organic Quinoa Pasta comes in a variety of shapes; my personal preferences are the thinner styles, such as vermicelli or angel hair, which cook more quickly.

Ancient Harvest Organic Quinoa Pasta

Available: Whole Foods

Organic Brown Rice Pasta Fusilli is another staple option.

Available: Trader Joe's

Explore Asian authentic cuisine is a new brand to the shelves. I prefer the Organic Thai Red Rice Pasta, which comes in several varieties, including elbow and thin vermicelli style. It's quite good. Other flavors include Organic Adzuki Bean Spaghetti. Available: Whole Foods

Pearl Barley: This delicious grain is high in fiber and niacin, which protects the cardiovascular system and lowers the risk of Type II diabetes. Barley is known for reducing cholesterol and protecting intestinal health, for decreasing the risk of colon cancer, and for helping to prevent gallstones and hemorrhoids. It also provides food for the good bacteria in the large intestine. I often combine 50% rice with 50% barley, as these grains cook at the same rate. Enjoy barley in soups, or for breakfast have a bowl with some pink Himalayan sea salt, goat butter and rainbow pepper. My favorite brand is Arrowhead Mills.

Available: www.HealthyLivingWithDeirdre.com/Marketplace & Whole Foods

Legumes / Beans

Black Beans: Like other legumes, the black bean's potassium, folate, vitamin B6 and phyto-nutrient content, along with flavonoids, support heart health. The high fiber content supports the lower intestinal tract, thereby lowering the risk of colon cancer. Recent research links bean intake to a lower risk of Type II diabetes, many types of cardiovascular disease, and several types of cancer.

Cooking tip: Soak beans in alkaline water overnight to reduce the cooking time. Drain the beans before cooking. I water plants with the discarded water. Alternately, you can sprout the beans by soaking them for a few days until they crack open. Remember to change the water twice day.

Serving suggestion: Add black beans to soup salads and salsa. Black beans are also a nice visual contrast on the plate when combined with a bit of yellow corn, diced red peppers and parsley.

Available: Whole Foods

Chick Peas/
Garbanzo Beans: Chick peas, also known as garbanzo beans, are, like most legumes, a great source of fiber. There are basic types of garbanzo beans: the common cream-colored ones usually found in a can are the "kabuli-type." And the other one is a "desi-type," a bit smaller and color range is from cream to black. As always, the darker the color the more powerful the nutrients! These heart-healthy beans help blood fat regulation and lower levels of LDL-cholesterol, total cholesterol, and triglycerides. Recent studies have shown that garbanzo bean fiber can be metabolized by bacteria in the colon to produce short chain fatty acids (SCFAs). These SCFAs fuel the cells of the intestinal wall, thereby lowering risk of colon cancer. Many public health organizations, including the American Diabetes Association, the American Heart Association, and the American Cancer Society, recommend legumes for preventing disease and opti-mizing health. Garbanzo beans, among other nutrients, contain more concentrated supplies of antioxidant phytonutrients and flavonoids.

Serving suggestion: Garbanzo bean salad: using cooked beans, mix in fresh squeezed lemon juice with extra virgin olive oil, finely chopped garlic, lots of flat Italian parsley and pink Himalayan sea salt to taste– it's yummy!

Available: Whole Foods

Kidney Beans:
Kidney beans come in white and different shades of red. As always, seek the darkest, richest colors for their high impact nutritional benefits. This legume is very high in protein and stabilizes blood sugars. Kidney beans are also rich in fiber, vitamins and minerals, including, iron, copper, folate and molybdenum, which is necessary to detoxify sulfates from the body. (Sulfates are a preservative commonly added to prepared foods.) Kidney beans also contain thiamin, which is important for brain function and memory retention. A study published in the *Archives of Internal Medicine* confirms that eating high fiber foods, such as kidney beans, helps prevent heart disease. When researchers analyzed data in relation to the risk of death from heart disease, they found that higher legume consumption was associated with a whopping 82% reduction in risk!

Kidney beans, like other beans, are also rich in soluble and insoluble fiber. Soluble fiber forms a gel-like substance in the digestive tract that binds with bile (which contains cholesterol) and ferries it out of the body. Research studies have shown that insoluble fiber not only helps to prevent constipation, but also helps prevent digestive disorders, such as irritable bowel syndrome and diverticulosis. Never consume raw kidney beans, because they contain high amounts of a potentially toxic substance called phytohaemagglutinin. This substance has been shown to disrupt cellular metabolism.

Serving suggestion: When preparing rice, add some kidney beans along with the vegetables.

Available: Whole Foods

Brown Rice Medley:

This is a nice precooked blend offered by Trader Joe's. If you leave it in alkaline water overnight, it will be edible in the morning without any cooking. This is a must have staple if you are in an area where you might lose electricity and not be able to cook! It also contains daikon radish seeds, which are tasty and satisfying. Since much of the mix is brown rice, this mix needs to be balanced with lots of vegetables. Try adding some sautéed onions, garlic and celery, and perhaps add a bit of steamed broccoli. Garnish with some parsley, and enjoy!

Cooking Tip: Sauté veggies in unflavored coconut oil and add vegetable bullion to the rice.

Available: Trader Joe's

Mahogany Rice:

This is a type of whole grain red rice that is high in fiber. Mahogany rice has a nutty flavor and is very rich in minerals and nutrients, including potassium, iron, manganese, magnesium, phosphorus and zinc. It contains powerful antioxidants called flavonoids; the darker the color, the more flavonoids in the food.

Serving suggestion: Toss in some pearl barley, sautéed vegetables, garnish with fresh herbs and enjoy.

My favorite brand is Lundberg.

Available: www.HealthyLivingWithDeirdre.com/Mark etplace & Whole Foods

Quinoa:

Quinoa has become a popular superfood and comes in three colors: white (or cream), black and red. Commonly considered a grain, it's actually a seed. Quinoa is packed with plant-based protein fiber, copper, iron, zinc, magnesium, manganese and folate, and vitamins B1, B2 and B6. NASA scientists have been looking at quinoa as a potentially suitable crop to be grown in outer space, mostly based on quinoa's high nutrient content, ease of use, and it cooks in 15 minutes, unlike other grains that take much longer. Genghis Khan fed his army on quinoa, a lightweight grain, packed with nutrition. Quinoa is my daughter's favorite breakfast food. She enjoys it with a basil pesto sauce. My favorite brand is Trader Joe's Organic White Quinoa because it comes in a resalable bag and is easy for my daughter to manage.

Available: Trader Joe's

The Extras:

You may have noticed that we do not discuss much about meat, poultry and seafood in this book. Same things apply. Eat less, grow your own, buy from the Amish, or as a last resort, buy organic, grass feed, antibiotic free and hormone free if you must. Use animal products less than you use salt or pepper. Dare to try it for 30 days and see how you feel! Also, be mindful that just because the package says no antibiotics does not mean the animal has not been administered other drugs. "Cage free" still does not mean that the animals are free to roam outside. Also, there are no factory farms or regular farms that offer a sanitation system for livestock, so the animal waste is seeping into the ground water and contaminating and polluting

> "There is a reason you take your kids to pick apples, but don't take them to the slaughterhouse."
> – humanefacts.org

our waterways at an alarming rate. As a population we are consuming way too many animal products. Simultaneously, farmers are finding ways to deliver more animals to market faster to increase their own profits. Again, voting with your dollar makes a difference! Make your vote count.

The best choice when selecting fish is fresh, whole sardines. And yes, consume the bones and all! If you like eating chicken, eat the black bone or ebony kind–found in Asian communities—who by culture boil the bird, toss the meat and eat the broth, as it has antibacterial properties in the bone marrow. When you choose to eat meat in restaurants, and organic options are not available, lamb is likely a better choice.

When it comes to cold cuts, hot dogs, sausages, try to forget they exist. Your body will be much happier. If you are weaning yourself off sandwich meats, try Applegate Farms. This is an organic line and the best in the marketplace. When making sandwiches with meat, consider removing the bread. Instead, roll the sliced meats into Boston or romaine lettuce leaves, with the meat on the top so that the meat is inside the roll.

Applegate Farms Sliced Deli Meats & Cheeses:
Available: Whole Foods

Daily Water Usage based on Diet
Vegan: 300 Gallons
Vegetarian: 1,200 Gallons
Meat-Eater 4,000 Gallons
Source: Mercy for Animals

Highlights to Remember:

The 80/20 Rule: you don't have to be perfect; simply do your best, relax and enjoy, explore and listen to your wonderful body.

A Dozen Tips And Take Aways!

When purchasing prepared foods or condiments:

1. Always read ingredients lists.

2. Beware of Advertising; truly nutritious foods most often will not have the words "healthy" or "natural" on the packaging.

3. Organic is better, yet still read the ingredients to prevent yourself from choosing foods with chemicals, additives, and health-hurting oils.

4. Avoid canola oil, (rapeseed oil,) dairy, sugars and soy in all possible ingredient list forms, preservatives, wheat, GMO's, aluminum chloride, and nearly 10,000 food additives.

5. Eat every color every day, especially blue, indigo and purple!

6. Upgrade your pantry with recommended products, fresh foods, herbs, spices and beverages.

7. Be sure to enjoy chocolate and Chile Peppers, the "happy foods."

8. Eat more rainbow foods and less animal products.

9. Eat more raw and fresh and less processed foods.

10. Enjoy your Plant and Pray Garden and Join A CSA Organic Farm.

11. Drink and cook with alkaline water and detox by juicing.

12. Get back to basics with your kitchen equipment.

Notables:

My Background And Perspective On Medical Studies:

I have mentioned quite a few studies throughout the book. Here is my intuitive and common sense understanding of the limitations of studies. One problem with studies is they are limited in duration, and therefore, don't bear the test of time. Additionally, studies are often funded by interested parties who intend a particular outcome, or more precisely "benefit" from a particular outcome.

Also noteworthy is that scientists and researchers often do you not have an intended outcome and are more neutral then the parties funding the study. However, much scientific work rarely gets published, and more rarely is exposed to the masses unless the company that benefits from the study provides research dollars to support it.

Largely because of the aforementioned factors, there is nothing more valuable than time to provide accuracy and perspective. In other words, the food or product or process is safe if it has been used for thousands of years and hasn't materially changed in any way. Recently, paleoanthropologists found bits of date stuck in the teeth of a 40,000-year-old Neanderthal. There's evidence that several of the fruits we enjoy eating today have been around for millennia in much the same form. For example, archaeologists have uncovered evidence of 780,000-year-old figs at a site in Northern Israel, as well as olives, plums, and pears from the Paleolithic era.

Source:
http://www.slate.com/articles/life/explainer/2012/02/the_real_cave man_diet_what_did_people_eat_in_prehistoric_times_.html

Of course, many of the products we consume today are far different than those consumed 300 years ago. It's therefore impossible to state the long-term effects brought upon ourselves and our children and our grandchildren and all future generations.

As a business owner, I respect and understand some of what it takes for businesses to bring new products to market quickly. If it's not profitable, it doesn't make any economic sense to do research and develop ideas and concepts into new products. Unfortunately, it is the profit motive itself that can make a guinea pig out of the unknowledgeable consumer. Those of us who are parents, or future parents, know that we are not only making choices for ourselves, but for our children, and perhaps for generations to come.

People, historically and presently, accept food and food practices that are part of our social fabric. Eating highly processed foods, and engaging in cooking methods that are questionable—such as the frequent use of the microwaves—is part and parcel of our society and our culture. However, that alone does not make them beneficial for us and our children. Microwaves may or may not be safe; and like many other modern choices that we make, the truth won't be known for many years, until the effects creep up on us, or on our children, and on future generations.

Here's my simple tip: if it was consumed 1000 years ago or cooked on a fire, in an iron pan or in a clay pot, hundreds or thousands of years ago, it's probably safe. If it's a newfangled Franken food ("Franken food" is the name for foods that contain ingredients the FDA approved, such as food additives) or a new cooking device, and it hasn't yet been tested on your grandchildren, we are smart to question its safety. Remember when the tobacco companies said there was nothing unsafe about cigarettes?

Here is a story I've been waiting 40 years to tell that brings this message home.

When I was in high school, friends of mine experienced menstrual issues, cramps and bloating and the like. To quash the pain and discomfort, they took analgesics, including ibuprofen, known by the brand names Advil and Midol.

Because my friends knew I was an avid reader when it came to health, they often consulted with me. I remember telling them, "Your body is giving you an early warning sign that something is out of balance. It's always best to identify the imbalance and correct it, rather than take a pill to mask it."

A citizen petition filed on Tuesday, Feb. 15, 2005 in Washington urges the government to require warning labels on ibuprofen products, such as Advil ®, Motrin ® and Aleve ®. The petition claims that ibuprofen can cause two potentially fatal reactions: Stevens-Johnson Syndrome and toxic epidermal necrolysis.

According to the National Kidney Foundation, "Many analgesics should not be used if there is decreased kidney function, because they reduce the blood flow to the kidney. Also, long term use with higher doses may harm normal kidneys and higher dosages with continual use may create kidney damage." Additionally, ibuprofen has been linked to a side effect known as "leaky gut syndrome" (LGS) because it may allegedly result in upper gastrointestinal bleeding.

The National Institute of Health (NIH) has already issued a warning about the possible ibuprofen side effects: "NSAIDs such as ibuprofen may cause ulcers, bleeding, or holes in the stomach or intestine. These problems may develop at any time during treatment, may happen without warning symptoms, and may cause death."

How did I, as a teenager, know about the dangers of ibuprofen? At the time, I was reading two ancient texts that I found in a second hand shop. To this day, they remain my most cherished books and reside on the bookshelf at my home, the content of which felt intuitively correct. I have read those books cover to cover many times over. Inexplicably, I felt as if I was remembering what I had already known!

Here's more about the two texts.

The Yellow Emperor's Classic of Internal Medicine is an ancient treatise on health and disease, said to have been written by the famous Chinese emperor, Huangdi around 2600 BC. The book, *Chinese Medical Herbs,* transcribed by Pen Ts'ao from *The Compendium of Materia Medica*, by Li Shizhen, is the most comprehensive medical book ever written in the history of traditional Chinese medicine. It lists all the plants, animals, minerals, and other items that were believed to have medicinal properties. The text consists of 1,892 entries.

Conclusion:

Did you enjoy this book? Did you learn something? Have you tried some of the recommended products?

Please share your honest feedback on Amazon.
I'd be grateful for your review!

Additionally, if you are consuming something that you are craving and you know is not working well for you and you'd like a recommendation on an upgrade email me at:

support@HealthyLivingWithDeirdre.com

A Personal Letter From Deirdre:

Dear Reader:

Thank you for reading and considering the contents of this book. We all do the best we can with what we have to work with. Remember to learn every day. Be mindful, and question everything! Find your personal intuitive common sense. Listen and communicate with your wonderful body, especially when it's communicating in the language of symptoms. Be sure you are always doing the best you can, just as you ask your children to do their best. Make better choices every day. As each of us takes one small, mindful step at a time, each and every day, our homes, our communities, and the planet we all share will be a happy and healthier place to live!

Perhaps most important in these confusing times, have faith in yourself and others!

Many Blessings,
Deirdre

ABOUT THE AUTHOR

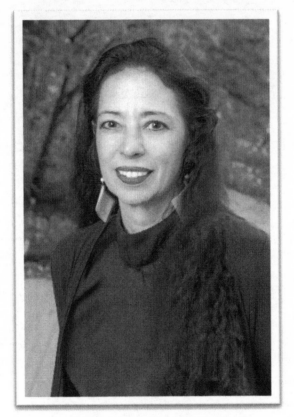

Deirdre Ventura, CHB, HHC

Deirdre is a mother and the owner and creator of The Harbor Rose, an eco-friendly, organic, non-toxic lifestyle lodging prototype that combines Deirdre's Hospitality Real Estate knowledge with her vast knowledge of health and wellness.

As a vegetarian with a personal commitment to health and wellness, she continues to acquire nutritional knowledge. In 2005, she graduated from the Institute of Integrative Nutrition as a Holistic Health Counselor. She is a Board Certified member of American Association of Drugless Practitioners. Her background in Chinese and Homeopathic Medicine has proved very helpful to her family, friends and clients.

Owner of Innvest Hotel Brokers, Deirdre has closed hundreds of hotel sales for banks, government agencies, hotel companies, REIT's and individuals. The firm, with over 40 years' experience, was named 2007 Top Hotel Broker by Hotel & Motel Management, which ranked Innvest, based on transaction volume, number fourteen nationwide. Hotel Brokers International (HBI) recognized her with numerous awards, including *"2002 Broker of the Year"* for the most transactions and highest dollar volume, and Salesperson of the Year.

A former HBI Board of Directors member, she co-chaired the committee that developed the Certified Hotel Broker Program. The CHB program is sponsored by Cornell University and HBI.

Deirdre has handled every type of hotel brokerage transaction imaginable, including sales, net leases, mortgage financing, sale-leasebacks; in 2002 alone she closed $80M in new construction transactions.

END NOTES

Chapter 1

Cohn, Barbara A., Wolff, Mary S., Cirillo, Pierra M. and Sholtz, Robert I. "DDT and Breast Cancer in Young Women: New Data on the Significance of Age at Exposure." *Environmental Health Perspectives.* National Institute of Environmental Health Sciences, n.d. Web. 01 Apr. 2016.

Miller, Kelli. "Cancer Risk Lingers for Long-Banned DDT." WebMD, n.d. Web. 01 Apr. 2016.

Healy, Melissa. Study Says Early DDT Exposure May Set up Females for Obesity, Diabetes. *Los Angeles Times*, 31 July 2014. Web. 01 Apr. 2016.

Karey, E., and La Frano, M. Newman, J., Moshier,E., Lindtner,C, Buettner, C. et al. "Pesticide DDT Linked to Slow Metabolism, Obesity and Diabetes." http://www.stonehearthnewsletters.com/30 July 2014.

El-Wakeil, N., Shalaby, S. Gehan Abdou, G. and Sallam, A. "Pesticide-Residue Relationship and Its Adverse Effects on Occupational Workers." Insecticides - Development of Safer and More Effective Technologies (2013): n. page. Web.

J, Dich, Zahm, SH. Hanberg A, and Adami HO. "Result Filters." National Center for Biotechnology Information. U.S. National Library of Medicine, n.d. Web. 01 Apr. 2016.

Lupkin, Sydney. "The Health Effects of GMO Foods." ABC News Network, 24 Apr. 2014. Web. 01 Apr. 2016.

BeWellBuzz. "Truth About Pesticides and GMO." N.p., 25 Sept. 2010. Web. 01 Apr. 2016.

Rappoport, Jon. "Why GMO Labeling Really Failed in Washington State: Stop Whining." Jim Marrs. N.p., n.d. Web. 01 Apr. 2016.

Perkins, Sharon. "Risks & Side Effects of Genetically Modified Food." Live Strong.com. 31 May 2015. Web. 01 Apr. 2016.

Rusiecki, J., Patel,R. Koutros,S, Beane-Freeman, L., Langren, O, Bonner, C., Lubin, M.R., Blair, J., Hoppin, A., and Michael C.R. "Cancer Incidence among Pesticide Applicators Exposed to Permethrin in the Agricultural Health Study." Environmental Health Perspectives. National Institute of Environmental Health Sciences, n.d. Web. 18 Mar. 2016

Arcury,T.A., Quant, S.A. Barr, D.B., Hoppin, J.A., McCauley, L., Grzywacz, J.G., Robson, M.G., "Farmworker Exposure to Pesticides: Methodologic Issues for the Collection of Comparable Data." - Environmental Health Perspectives. June 2006.

Curwin, B.D., Hein, M.J., Sanderson,W.T., Striley, C., Heederik, D., Kromhout, Reynolds,H.S.J., and Alavanja,M.C. "Urinary Pesticide Concentrations Among Children, Mothers and Fathers Living in Farm and Non-Farm Households in Iowa." Annals of Occupational Hygiene 51.1 (2006): 53-65. Web.

Kaefer, Christine M. "Herbs and Spices in Cancer Prevention and Treatment." U.S. National Library of Medicine, n.d. Web. 18 Mar. 2016.
"Lee KJ, et al. (2007). "Coffee Consumption and Risk of Colorectal Cancer in a Population-based Prospective Cohort of

Japanese Men and Women." Int J Cancer;121:1312-8, Web. 18 Mar. 2016.

Carman, Judy. "Evidence of GMO Harm in Pig Study." Sustainable Pulse. N.p., 11 June 2013. Web. 18 Mar. 2016.

"Gmo's Unfit for Consumption - More Evidence." HotCopper. N.p., n.d. Web. 18 Mar. 2016.

Carman, J. "32% of Pigs on a GM Diet Had a Higher Rate of Severe Stomach Inflammation; so Screen GM-fed Pork Eaters?" *Journal of Organic Systems.* 13 June 2013.

Reiss, R. Johnston, J., Tucker, K., Desesso, J.M., and Keen, C.L. "Estimation of Cancer Risks and Benefits Associated with a Potential Increased Consumption of Fruits and Vegetables." *Food and Chemical Toxicology* 50.12 (2012): 4421-427.

Gilles, E.S., Clair,E, Mesnage, R., Gress, S. Defarge, N. Malatesta,M., Hennequin,D., and Spiroux de Vendômois, J. "Criigen: GM Maize and Roundup Can Cause Tumours, Multiple Organ Damage and Premature Death." GMO EVIDENCE. N.p., n.d. Web. 18 Mar. 2016.

Chapter 2

Lava, Neil D. "Controversial Claims About the Causes of Alzheimer's Disease." Controversial Alzheimer's Disease Risk Factors. WebMD, n.d. Web. 01 Apr. 2016.

O'Connor, Anahad. "BPA Lurks in Canned Soups and Drinks." Well BPA Lurks in Canned Soups and Drinks Comments. N.p., 22 Nov. 2011. Web. 01 Apr. 2016.

Sifferlin, Alexandra. "How BPA May Disrupt Brain Development." TIME.com 26 Feb. 2013.

Huber, Colleen. "Effects of Bisphenol A and a Potential Link to Alzheimer's." N.p., n.d. Web. 01 Apr. 2016.

BPA-Free Does Not Mean Safe. Most Plastics Leach Hormone-Disrupting Chemicals. My Plastic Free Life, N.p., 12 Apr. 2011.

http://greenopedia.com/alkaline-acid-food-chart/
http://www.energiseforlife.com/acid-alkaline-food-chart-1.1.pdf

King, Margie. "Miso Protects Against Radiation, Cancer and Hypertension." N.p., 20 Aug. 2013. Web. 01 Apr. 2016.

Adams, Mike. "The Astonishing Radioprotective Effects of MISO Explained: Nagasaki, Hiroshima and Chernobyl Survivors Speak Out... Eat to Live!" NaturalNews. N.p., 19 May 2015. Web. 01 Apr. 2016.

Marcola, Joseph. "The Truth About Soy Foods: Can Soy Damage Your Health?" N.p., 18 Sept. 2010. Web. 01 Apr. 2016.

Terrain, Mary Vance. "The Dark Side of Soy." N.p., Aug. 2007. Web. 01 Apr. 2016.

http://www.westonaprice.org/soy-alert/

Kerr, Gord. "What Are the Dangers of Soy Lecithin Ingestion?" LIVESTRONG.COM. 16 Aug. 2013. Web. 01 Apr. 2016.

Bell, JM, and Lundberg, PK. "Effects of a Commercial Soy Lecithin Preparation on Development of Sensorimotor Behavior and Brain Biochemistry in the Rat." U.S. National Library of Medicine, 18 Jan. 1985. Web. 01 Apr. 2016.

Kerr, Michael, Valencia Higuera, and Butler, Natalie. "Soy Allergy." N.p., 1 July 2015. Web. 01 Apr. 2016. www.NaturalNews.com.

Chapter 3

Veracity, Dani. "Asthma Explained by Common Allergy to Milk and Dairy Products." Natural News, 4 Aug. 2005. Web. 01 Apr. 2016.

Annigan, Jan. "Dairy & the Human Digestive System." N.p., n.d. Web. 01 Apr. 2016.

Schwartzmann, Laura. "Food Allergy Labels Too Vague." CBS Interactive, 15 Sept. 2008. Web. 01. Apr. 2016.

Chapter 4

Blodget, Henry. "CHART OF THE DAY: American Per-Capita Sugar Consumption Hits 100 Pounds Per Year." Business Insider. 19 Feb. 2012.

Null, Gary. "Sugar: Killing Us Sweetly. Staggering Health Consequences of Sugar on Health of Americans." *Global Research Journals,* 13 Mar. 2014. Web. 01 Apr. 2016.

Klamer, Holly. "High Sugar Side Effects." LIVESTRONG.COM. 13 Feb. 2011. Web. 01 Apr. 2016.

Chapter 6

Gray, Richard. "Cancer and Psychiatric Drugs Found in Tap Water." SOTT.net. N.p., 13 Jan. 2008. Web. 01 Apr. 2016.

Feature, Kathleen. "Drugs in Our Drinking Water?" WebMD. 10 Mar. 2008. Web. 01 Apr. 2016.

"Study Finds Traces of Drugs in Drinking Water in 24 Major U.S. Regions. FOX News Network, 10 Mar. 2008. Web. 01 Apr. 2016.

Goodman, Amy. "Sedatives and Sex Hormones in Our Water Supply." Alternet. N.p., 25 Mar. 2008. Web. 01 Apr. 2016.

Cloherty, Megan. "What is in the Potomac River's Water?" WTOP. N.p., 29 May 2013. Web. 03 Apr. 2016.

Klatell, James. "'Intersex' Fish Spark Pollution Debate." CBSNews. CBS Interactive, 6 Sept. 2006. Web. 03 Apr. 2016.

"Probe: Pharmaceuticals in Drinking Water." CBSNews. CBS Interactive, 10 Mar. 2008. Web. 03 Apr. 2016.

Chapter 7

"Archives of Internal Medicine." Journal Impact Factor & Description. N.p., n.d. Web. 19 Mar. 2016.

"Result Filters." National Center for Biotechnology Information. U.S. National Library of Medicine, n.d. Web. 19 Mar. 2016.

Sessoms, Gail. "Purple Foods List." LIVESTRONG.COM. 10 Jan. 2014. Web. 03 Apr. 2016.

Helm, Janet. "Purple Veggies Show Promising Health Benefits." Chicago Tribune. 19 Apr. 2009. Web. 03 Apr. 2016.

"Epidemiology and Genomics Research Program." Usual Dietary Intakes: NHANES Food Frequency Questionnaire (FFQ). N.p., n.d. Web. 19 Mar. 2016.

Chapter 8

Kaur, M., Agarwal, C., and Agarwal, R. "Anticancer and Cancer Chemopreventive Potential of Grape Seed Extract and Other Grape-Based Products." The Journal of Nutrition. Sept. 2009. Web. 03 Apr. 2016.

Thomas, John. "Blindness, Mad Cow Disease and Canola Oil." N.p., Mar. 1996. Web.

Milligan, Albert T. "Dangers of Cooking with Canola Oil." MyoneSourcecom. N.p., 2 Nov. 2011. Web. 03 Apr. 2016.

Chapter 9

Kim, Steve. "Herbs to Lower Blood Pressure." Healthline. N.p., 20 Jan. 2016. Web. 03 Apr. 2016.

Pravel, Donna Earnest. "Holy Basil Is a Clinically Proven Antioxidant, Cancer Fighter, Neuropathy Healer, and Anti-microbial."NaturalNews. 5 Feb. 2012. Web. 03 Apr. 2016.

Cass, Hyla. "Can Cinnamon Fight Cancer? Life Enhancement Magazine, Jan. 2006. Web. 03 Apr. 2016.

Baker, William L., Gutierrez, Gabriella, White, Michael, and Kluger. "Diabetes Care." Effect of Cinnamon on Glucose Control and Lipid Parameters. N.p., 28 Sept. 2007. Web. 03 Apr. 2016.

http://cancerpreventionresearch.aacrjournals.org/content/8/5/444.abstract

http://www.ncbi.nlm.nih.gov/pubmed/19473851

Lorentzen, Karin. "Cinnamon Research Holds Promise for Colorectal Cancer Prevention."UANews. Arizona.edu. N.p., n.d. 8 June, 2015.

"Postharvest Quality and Safety in Fresh-cut Vegetables and Fruits - UNIVERSITY OF ARIZONA." Postharvest Quality and Safety in Fresh-cut Vegetables and Fruits - UNIVERSITY OF ARIZONA. N.p., n.d. Web. 19 Mar. 2016.

Sass, Cynthia. "5 Sweet Health Benefits of Cinnamon." Real Simple. N.p., n.d. Web. 19 Mar. 2016.

Daniells, Stephen. "Chili Could Boost Insulin Control, Says Study." NutraIngredients.com. N.p., 24 July 2006. Web. 03 Apr. 2016.

MacLean CH, Newberry SJ, Mojica WA, Khanna P, Issa AM, Suttorp MJ, Lim YW, Traina SB, Hilton L, Garland R, Morton SC. "Effects of omega-3 fatty acids on cancer risk: a systematic review." JAMA. 2006 Apr 26;295(16):1900.

Mori A, Lehmann S, O'Kelly J, Kumagai T, Desmond JC, Pervan M, McBride WH, Kizaki M,and Koeffler HP."Capsaicin, a Component of Red Peppers, Inhibits the Growth of Androgen-

Independent, P53 Mutant Prostate Cancer Cells." Cancer Res. 2016.

Larsson, SC, Bergkvist, L., and Wolk, A. "Consumption of Sugar and Sugar-sweetened Foods and the Risk of Pancreatic Cancer in a Prospective Study." *The American Journal of Clinical Nutrition.* "Web. 19 Mar. 2016.

Radulian, G., Rusu, E. Dragomir, A., and Posea, M. "The Insulin Index." Diabetes Developments RSS. N.p., n.d. Web. 19 Mar. 2016.

Tillet, T. "Carcinogenic Crops: Analyzing the Effect of Aflatoxin on Global Liver Cancer Rates." *Environmental Health Perspectives Journal.* June 2010.

Remos, MI, Allen, LH, Mangas, DM, Jagust, W.J., Haan, MN, Green, R. Miller, JW. "Low folate status is associated with impaired cognitive function and dementia in the Sacramento Area Latino Study on Aging." *American Journal of Clinical Nutrition,* 2005 Dec.

Alper, Corinna M., Mattes, Richard D. "Peanut Consumption Improves Indices of Cardiovascular Disease Risk in Healthy Adults." *Journal of American College of Nutrition,* March, 2003.

Chapter 10

Campbell, T. Colin, Campbell, M. Thomas. *The China Study: Startling Implications for Diet, Weight Loss and Long Term-Health.* BenbBella Books.

Chapter 11

Belluck, Pam. "To Improve a Memory, Consider Chocolate." The New York Times. 26 Oct. 2014. Web. 03 Apr. 2016.

Hammit, Lauren. "Cocoa Flavanols Improve Vascular and Blood Pressure Measures for Coronary Artery Disease Patients." UC San Francisco. Web.06, July, 2010

Fraga, Cesar G. "Cocoa, Diabetes, and Hypertension: Should We Eat More Chocolate?" The American Journal of Clinical Nutrition. Web. 19 Mar. 2016.

"Cocoa, The Health Miracle | Medicine Hunter." Medicine Hunter.com.Web. 19 Mar. 2016

Chapter 12

"BBC NEWS | Health | Green Tea Cuts Fatal Illness Risk." BBC News. BBC, 12 Sept. 2006. Web. 03 Apr. 2016.
green tea increases the metabolism and burns fat
"Green Tea Extract 500mg Capsules (100 Capsules)." True Nutrition. N.p., n.d. Web. 19 Mar. 2016.

"The Top Fat-Burning Foods." Health.com. N.p., n.d. Web. 19 Mar. 2016.

"Green Tea Fat-Burning Phenomenon: The Secret Behind It All!"Bodybuilding.com. N.p., 30 Jan. 2008. Web. 19 Mar. 2016.

"Green Tea Metabolism - Boost Metabolism 101." Boost Metabolism 101. N.p., 27 Aug. 2015. Web. 19 Mar. 2016.

"Melt Flab Away: The Best Fat Burning Foods." Cosmopolitan. N.p., 27 May 2014. Web. 19 Mar. 2016.

Chapter 13

Mao, D. "Kidney Bean." Askdr.mao.com/natral-health-dictionary/kidney-bean Arnarson, Atli. "Kidney Beans 101: Nutrition Facts and Health Benefits." RSS 20. N.p., Mar. 2016. Web. 03 Apr. 2016.

Tremblay, Sylvie. "Nutrients & Benefits of Chick Peas and Garbanzo Beans." Web. 03 Apr. 2016.

Hendrick, Bill. "Black Rice Is Cheap Way to Get Antioxidants." WebMD, 26 Aug. 2010. Web. 03 Apr. 2016.

"The Brown Rice Cleanse." Just Cleansing RSS. N.p., n.d. Web. 03 Apr. 2016.

"The Forbidden Rice: Black Rice Nutrition & Benefits." Dr Axe. N.p., 08 Feb. 2015. Web. 03 Apr. 2016.
Nair, Priya. "Health Benefits of Red Lentils." Value Food. N.p., 26 Feb. 2014. Web. 03 Apr. 2016

Walsh, Caley. "The 10 Healthiest Foods: Red Lentils." Favehealthyrecipes.com. N.p., 2 Mar. 2009. Web. 03 Apr. 2016.

"AICR's Foods That Fight Cancer™." AICR All. N.p., 17 May 2013. Web. 03 Apr. 2016.

INDEX